Medicine
and Health
in Africa

Medicine and Health in Africa

MULTIDISCIPLINARY PERSPECTIVES

EDITED BY
Paula Viterbo
Kalala Ngalamulume

MICHIGAN STATE UNIVERSITY PRESS | *East Lansing* ∎ LIT VERLAG | *Münster*

☉ The paper used in this publication meets the minimum requirements of ANSI/NISO Z39.48-1992 (R 1997) (Permanence of Paper).

LIT Verlag
Münster

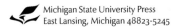 Michigan State University Press
East Lansing, Michigan 48823-5245

Printed and bound in the United States of America.

17 16 15 14 13 12 11   1 2 3 4 5 6 7 8 9 10

LIBRARY OF CONGRESS CATALOGING-IN-PUBLICATION DATA
Medicine and health in Africa : multidisciplinary perspectives / edited by Paula Viterbo and Kalala Ngalamulume.
p. ; cm.
Includes bibliographical references and index.
ISBN 978-0-87013-991-8 (pbk. : alk. paper) — ISBN 978-3-8258-9226-5 (pbk. : alk. paper) 1. Public health—Africa. 2. Health policy—Africa. I. Viterbo, Paula. II. Ngalamulume, Kalala J.
[DNLM: 1. Public Health—Africa. 2. Acquired Immunodeficiency Syndrome—Africa. 3. Developing Countries—Africa. 4. HIV Infections—Africa. 5. Health Policy—Africa. 6. Malaria—Africa. WA 395]
RA545.M45 2011
362.1096—dc22
2010033514

Cover design by Sharp Des!gns, Inc.
Book design by Lit Verlag
Cover: Yourba maternity figure with offering bowl, Nigeria (early 20th c.). Wood, iron, pigment.
Bryn Mawr College – Special Collections – BMC. 99.5.7

g **green** Michigan State University Press is a member of the Green Press Initiative and is committed
press to developing and encouraging ecologically responsible publishing practices. For more
INITIATIVE information about the Green Press Initiative and the use of recycled paper in book publishing, please
visit *www.greenpressinitiative.org*.

■ Visit Michigan State University Press at *www.msupress.msu.edu*

CONTENTS

FOREWORD

Earlier versions of the articles in this book were presented at the Health and Medicine in Africa Workshop at Bryn Mawr and Haverford Colleges on April 13-15, 2005. The project grew out of a requirement of a Mellon Postdoctoral Fellowship, which I held at the Bryn Mawr Center for Science in Society (CIS) during the 2003-04 and 2004-05 school years. My initial intention was to invite one scholar to campus, to talk about some engaging and currently relevant aspect of the history of medicine in Africa. But to my amazement and delight, the first three possible speakers I contacted were all not only very eager to participate, but in turn referred other colleagues, who upon invitation enthusiastically joined the group. What started as a single talk quickly expanded, first into an afternoon of talks, then into a multi-day, and most exciting, multidisciplinary workshop. Clearly, there was a widespread interest and a felt need for a venue to discuss the complex issues in African health from an interdisciplinary perspective. Encouraged by everybody I talked to, especially Paul Grobstein, then CIS director, I started to look for ways to stretch the funding, originally planned for one speaker, into the resources necessary to cover a three-day workshop with more than twenty participants. My co-editor, Kalala Ngalamulume, from Bryn Mawr Africana Studies Program and Department of History helped with the grant application process, which also profited from the administrative expertise of Selene Platt, then CIS secretary. In the meantime, it also became clear that the workshop would benefit from the joint collaboration of our colleagues at Haverford, especially Kay Edwards, director of the Center for Peace & Global Citizenship, and Iruka Okeke, a biologist working on antimicrobial resistance in Africa. In the end, we owe the enormous success of the workshop to the generous support of the following organizations and departments (listed in decreasing order of financial contribution): the Mellon Tri-Co Fund (Bryn Mawr, Haverford, and Swarthmore Colleges), the

Center For International Studies at Bryn Mawr College, the Bryn Mawr College Center For Science in Society, the Haverford College Center For Peace & Global Citizenship, the Marian E. Koshland Integrated Natural Sciences Center at Haverford College, the Bryn Mawr College 1902 Fund, the Africana Studies Program at Haverford College, the Feminist & Gender Studies Program at Bryn Mawr College, and the Bryn Mawr College Department of History.

One of the papers presented at the workshop, and included in our collection, had been already published. Two other papers have since appeared elsewhere, as duly noted below. For the gracious permission to reprint them, we thank the editors of the *Population and Development Review*, *The Journal of World History*, and *Culture, Medicine and Psychiatry*.

PAULA VITERBO
DECEMBER 2007

Crystal Biruk is a doctoral candidate in anthropology at the University of Pennsylvania. She has been awarded Social Science Research Council (SSRC), Wenner Gren Foundation, and National Science Foundation (NSF) grants to conduct her dissertation research on the politics of the production of knowledge about AIDS in Malawi.

Laura McGough is currently finishing a book on the history of syphilis in Renaissance Venice. She teaches at the University of Ghana in Accra, and works as a consultant on HIV/AIDS projects in West Africa.

Kalala Ngalamulume is Associate Professor of Africana Studies and History at Bryn Mawr College. He is currently completing a book manuscript on the social history of medicine in colonial Saint-Louis-du-Senegal and is researching a book on the social history of leisure in Senegal. His research on teaching scholarship, on colonialism and social change in Congo/Zaire, and on colonial pathologies in Senegal has appeared in several scholarly journals.

Zolani Ngwane is Associate Professor of Anthropology at Haverford College. He is currently finishing a book manuscript on higher education in South Africa and pursuing research on the impact of HIV/AIDS on gender division of labor in household economies in rural South Africa.

Iruka Okeke is a microbiologist in the Department of Biology, Haverford College and a Branco Weiss Fellow of the Society in Science, Zürich. Her research focuses on the epidemiology, disease-causing mechanisms and drug resistance of bacteria. She is particularly interested in bacteria that cause childhood diarrhea, and in drug resistance in West Africa.

James Pfeiffer, an anthropologist and MPH, is Associate Professor in the Department of Health Services, School of Public Health and Community Medicine, at the University of Washington, Seattle. He is also Director of Mozambique Operations for Health Alliance International at its headquarters in Seattle, where he coordinates a wide range of projects on AIDS treatment. His work on Pentecostalism, AIDS, and health in Mozambique has received grants from the National Science Foundation, the Wenner-Gren Foundation, and the National Institutes of Health.

Judith Porter is a sociologist whose research specialty is AIDS and drug addiction. She is currently studying the role of syringe exchange programs as a bridge to services for heroin addicts. She is Research Professor of Sociology at Bryn Mawr College.

Jonathan Sadowsky is Theodore J. Castele Professor of the History of Medicine at Case Western Reserve University. His book *Imperial Bedlam: Institutions of Madness and Colonialism in Southwest Nigeria* was published by the University of California Press in 1999. He is currently working on a history of electroconvulsive therapy in the United States.

Evelyne Shuster, Ph.D. is a philosopher and the clinical ethicist in charge of the Ethics Program at the Department of Veterans Affairs Medical Center, Philadelphia, Pennsylvania.

Paula Viterbo is a historian of science and medicine currently finishing a book about the discovery of the woman's time of ovulation and the development of natural family planning in America. Her next project will focus on reproductive health in twentieth-century Portuguese colonies. She also works as a researcher in the Papers of Thomas Jefferson: Retirement Series, at Monticello.

Faith Wallace-Gadsden is a molecular microbiology graduate student at Tufts University Sackler School. Her research interests focus on bacterial pathogens that affect underdeveloped countries. She is currently studying

Vibrio cholerae isolated from patients in Bangladesh.

Susan Watkins is a professor in the Department of Sociology at the University of Pennsylvania and a Visiting Scientist at the California Center for Population Research, University of California, Los Angeles. Her research has been on demographic change in historical Europe and the United States, and more recently in sub-Saharan Africa.

James L.A. Webb, Jr. is a professor of history at Colby College who writes and teaches in the fields of world history, African history, environmental history, and historical epidemiology. He has recently finished a book manuscript on the global history of malaria entitled *Humanity's Burden* and is now engaged in a new project on the history of malaria in Africa from 1950 to 2010.

CHAPTER 1

Introduction

KALALA NGALAMULUME AND PAULA VITERBO

The present collection provides multidisciplinary perspectives on key health problems in Africa, and on the heavy burden they have exerted on its people. Most studies included here focus on the two major epidemics currently responsible for premature death in the African continent, namely AIDS and malaria. But as other chapters remind us, attention to these two infections should not come at the price of neglecting equally widespread problems, such as waterborne diseases and stigmatizing mental illnesses. To study these multiple health issues, the authors in this volume utilize different approaches, ranging from biological perspectives, essential to comprehend disease etiology or antimicrobial resistance, to contextual and social constructionist approaches, without which the understanding and amelioration of disease proves impossible.

The last two decades have witnessed a growing interest in the study of health and medicine in Africa in multiple academic fields, e.g. anthropology, biology, history, medical sciences (especially epidemiology, clinical medicine, and public health), and sociology. This varied body of work has contributed to our understanding of indigenous healing traditions,[1] colonial and missionary medicines,[2] medical ideologies,[3] and the medical professions.[4] But the main target of the recent scholarship has increasingly been the social, economic, and policy impact of HIV/AIDS on African societies. Indeed, these studies have explained the correlation between the disease's etiology and entrenched poverty, economic inequality, and the subordination of women,[5] between the representations of the epidemic and the politics of sexuality,[6] and between medical knowledge and theories about putative risk groups (homosexuals, sex workers, heroin users, army personnel, traders, truck drivers, migrant laborers, and refugees).[7]

Historians entered this debate, saw links between AIDS and bygone epidemics in Africa and elsewhere, and abandoning the profession's perennial fear of Whiggishness, even suggested health policies based on lessons from the past.[8] They pointed to "certain ideological and theoretical continuities"[9] of hegemonic medical discourse and representations, going back to the nineteenth century widespread perceptions of West and Central Africa as the "white man's grave."[10] At the time, yellow fever and malaria, responsible for high mortality rates within the European population, were constructed as the "white man's diseases," while cholera and plague were viewed as "the black man's diseases."[11] Such historical analyses underline the problematic nature of present interactions among science, medicine, social structures, culture, and power.

Health and Medicine in Africa builds and expands on the work mentioned above. The book responds to the felt need for a dialogue across disciplinary concerns and to the critical importance of bringing historical perspectives to our understanding of current health crises, of seeking in (successful as well as failed) past experiences explanations that may prove useful for the present. It also responds to earlier pleas for a careful examination, not of culture as an analytical category, but of the conditions under which diverse meanings produced by a particular culture proliferate,[12] for multidisciplinary approaches to understand disease production, and for the development of therapies involving the collaboration of experts, policy-makers, patients and their communities.[13] The contributors to this collection share the notion that conceptions of health and illness, as well as meanings of particular diseases, medicines, and healing practices are socially constructed and historically framed. We maintain that biomedical knowledge, in particular concerning the expansion of diagnostic categories, prognostic procedures, and disease classifications, is about contentious social negotiation, debate, controversy, and consensus building, and that, as Charles Rosenberg argued a while ago, the ways in which disease is framed can have specific behavioral and policy implications.[14] Many chapters in the present book go beyond the simple cultural explanations of the impact of particular diseases, to examine illness narratives, everyday practices, processes, and strategies of prevention not included in the traditional cultural norms.

This collection also underlines a political economy approach to health issues, which places disease within its social, economic, political, cultural, ideological, and historical contexts, when analyzing disease production, the functions of the medical professions, and the structural causes of patient inequality and vulnerability. As Jean Comaroff has shown, we need to bring together global and local perspectives in order to make sense of the experiences of a particular population.[15] An analysis of current health crises in Africa must take into account the consequences of colonial conquest, capitalist exploitation of wage laborers, the Cold War, the economic crisis, the Structural Adjustment Programs (SAPs) of the 1970s and 1980s, urban sprawl, civil wars, and gender inequities. These factors combine in different ways to determine the unequal social distribution of disease, that is, which groups of people get sick with which diseases.[16] Subscribing to this view, many of our contributions raise questions about the process of construction of medical knowledge itself. They argue against essentialist conceptions of history and culture embedded in official medical discourse and scholarship, the primacy of cultural explanations of disease etiologies, and the emphasis on behavioral paradigms at the expense of other, structural factors. This critical approach fosters innovative preventive strategies.

In a recent collection, Kalipeni *et al.* discuss the policy impact of media interpretations of the AIDS epidemic, which continue to reproduce the negative colonial images of Africa as a dark and diseased continent, and of Africans as ignorant, hypersexual, promiscuous and culturally backward. This work alerts us to the shortcomings of the dominant, ethnocentric, biomedical paradigms used to understand AIDS in Africa, and the inadequacy of top-down interventions to combat infection.[17] But despite this and other critiques, essentialist conceptions of culture and the blame-the-victim component of medical ideology have persisted. In a volume published last year, one author argues that the spread of the AIDS epidemic was mainly the result of "Nigerian culture," or, as he puts it, the "customs and social practices" within Nigeria's "traditional and religious frameworks," and in order to address the problem he suggests a strong program of "culture change."[18] The prominence of these notions in the media, movie industry, and scholarship has informed a particular construction of an "African AIDS" as primarily a product of culture rather than political economy. This view has policy implications, such as the investment on vaccine trials at the expense of treatments for opportunistic infections.[19]

Discussions in current scholarship have often obscured the distinction between short- and long-term changes in a given culture, especially in those societies that have experienced repeated episodes of structural break. On the one hand, those who call for "culture change" in fact pay attention only to the long-term continuity of the broad structure of a society, but ignore the continuous process of its small transformations under the pressure of colonialism, westernization, Christianization, urbanization, market forces, and war. On the other hand, one needs to keep in mind that the changeable, adaptive, individual intentions and behaviors constitutive of a culture are to some extent expressions of the hegemony of a particular, relatively stable structure of meaning over other alternatives.[20]

The authors in our collection recognize the role of cultural forces like polygyny, *lobola*, patriarchy, and widow inheritance in structuring human behavior, but they argue against the essentialist conceptions of African culture widespread in journalistic and scholarly discussions concerning the etiology and prevention of HIV/AIDS, which emphasize the role of cultural categories, norms, values, and ideologies, but neglect actors' motives and practices, and the specific realities of social inequality. As Crystal Biruk's study shows (chapter 2), the representation of widow inheritance by a male kin as the only possible risky practice responsible for the elevated rates of HIV infection among the Luo of western Kenya is misleading, does not take into account recent changes in the practice of widow inheritance, and turns the attention away from failed public health interventions or development agendas. Biruk persuasively shows that local narratives and perceptions of risk depict a far more complex situation.

By focusing solely on cultural categories and routinized meanings, scholars and policy-makers fail to realize that the mentalities of the people they study have undergone significant transformations. Thus, as Zolani Ngwane argues (chapter 3), we should focus on the actors' thoughts and actions that help understand the processes involved in the reproduction or change of structural features, that is, the specific kinds of actions involving pragmatic choices, strategizing, and norm manipulation. For Ngwane, the interesting questions are those that underline what the actors want, and what is materially useful for them within their changing cultural and historical context.

This approach is particularly useful when considering prevention. Susan Watkins' analysis of the local strategies of prevention formulated by men and women in Malawi (chapter 4) shows that rural communities have challenged the conventional prevention strategies (abstinence, fidelity, and condom use), and adopted innovative preventive strategies that provide reasons for optimism – reduction in the number of partner, partner selection based on local knowledge, divorce, and renewed religious commitment. In sum, instead of relying on the cultural models described by long-dead anthropologists and missionaries, the best way to understand the changes that have occurred in a given society is to be mindful of what people say and do.

How can we, otherwise, explain the failure of the policies implemented by international organizations in the fight against the AIDS global pandemic? For Evelyne Shuster (chapter 5), the problem stems from inadequacies of the four approaches to the disease used so far, namely the humanitarian, military, commercial and human rights models. She argues that, compared with the other models, the human rights model has the advantage of underlining the enforcement of laws against stigmatization and discrimination of HIV/AIDS patients, and of promoting health care, nutrition, education, gender equality, and employment. At least from a theoretical perspective, this seems to be the most adequate framework, since AIDS is above all an epidemic of inequality.

Interventions to reduce HIV/AIDS stigma play a crucial role in the success of preventive measures, such as HIV testing and dissemination of accurate information about the condition. Laura McGough's research (chapter 6) on past experiences with epidemics has shown that stigma associated with a sexually-transmitted disease does not end with the availability of treatment; instead, the stigma of infection often shifts from the majority of patients to scapegoats, that is, to the most vulnerable members of the society who cannot defend themselves, such as the poor and marginalized, females, foreigners, and outsiders. Judith Porter's sociological study (chapter 7) strongly suggests that the reduction of stigma encourages individuals to get tested for HIV.

The seriousness, novelty, and cultural connotations of the AIDS epidemic have led to its prominence as a topic of scholarly and media attention. And yet, malaria today kills more people than any other disease. In fact, it is responsible for more deaths, especially of children and adults with compromised immune systems, than at the time of the great anti-malaria campaigns of the 1950s and 1960s. Biomedical scholars have explained that the anti-malaria efforts undertaken five decades ago failed for multiple reasons. First, these efforts were aimed at eradicating the disease, an ambitious goal that could not be achieved; as years went by, public health authorities settled for the more realistic goal of disease control. Second, artificial barriers had developed between disease control specialists and health systems experts. Third, public health officials relied heavily on one or two interventions, especially DDT house-spray programs, which eventually contributed to insecticide resistance. Fourth, public health officials failed to approach malaria as a disease associated with poverty (as had been demonstrated in the American South).[21] Finally, malaria control programs, already underfunded, were not integrated in the mainstream health sector.[22] The spread of chloroquine resistance, combined with DDT's ineffectiveness,[23] called for a new cost-effective strategy to combat *Plasmodium falciparum* and its vectors.[24]

The inability of post-colonial governments to overcome or even tackle the burden of malaria underlies its continuous growth, making it the main killer in contemporary Africa. Resources continue to be squandered and dilapidated by corrupt officers, or simply diverted to other projects, including weapon purchases. To be true, the legacy of colonialism is not easy to surmount; during the early period, colonial states allocated priorities and health resources primarily to the protection of the health of European troops, civil servants, merchants, and Africans associated with them. But even if for arguable reasons, during the post-war period the colonial states spent more resources than the present governments on the improvement of living and working conditions of the Africans, including on malaria control programs. *Health and Medicine in Africa* brings an interdisciplinary approach to understanding the persistence and incidence of falciparum malaria on the continent. James Webb's ambitious synthesis (chapter 8) combines research findings from microbiology, archaeology, archaeobotany, and linguistics, which underline the interaction between genetic endowment, global environmental conditions, and socioeconomic factors. His study establishes a linkage among plantain and banana cultivation, sedentarization and endemic malarial infections. His model provides one of the best current understandings of the etiology of falciparum malaria and early population movements.

Health and Medicine in Africa also pays attention to two neglected, but all too real, health problems in Africa – antimicrobial resistance and mental illness. As Faith Wallace-Gadsden and Iruka Okeke document (chapter 9), the slow development of antimicrobials since the 1970s, combined with drug degradation and counterfeiting, resulted in increasing resistance to cheap, first-line drugs, rendering many infections untreatable, and adding to the economic burden of infectious diseases. The current main threat of this "hidden epidemic" comes from the malaria germ's resistance to chloroquine, but other germs responsible for diarrheal diseases, sexually-transmitted infections, tuberculosis, and a variety of respiratory illnesses have now also become resistant to first-line antibiotics. Thus there is an urgent need for the implementation of an effective resistance-control strategy.

Kalala Ngalamulume's research (chapter 10) adds to the meager body of work about mental illness in Africa. His study of mental illness in nineteenth-century Saint-Louis du Sénégal helps us understand the process of construction of racialized medical knowledge that lies at the roots of the established standards of normality/deviance, and morality/immorality. His approach goes beyond the binary opposition colonizer/colonized and the ways in which the French colonial authorities tried to regulate madness, to also include the illness experiences of French citizens in the colonial city, as well as the agency of the family in mediating custody for the mental patients.

This volume closes with two contributions that reflect on the current state of health and medicine in Africa, once again pointing to the collaboration of different disciplinary approaches in order to assure successful treatment outcomes. James Pfeiffer's study of the current practices of faith healing in Mozambique (chapter 11) shows the linkage between macro social processes (such as the Cold War, the Structural Adjustment Programs, and the commoditization of community life) and people's treatment choices. The illness narratives and surveys analyzed by Pfeiffer shed new light on the recent popularity of Pentecostalism (and the concomitant decline of traditional healing) in southern Africa, as a way for people to cope with ailments believed to have a spiritual cause.

If Pfeiffer's work underlines the fluidity of the health and disease arena in Africa, where rapid and often dramatic socioeconomic changes require people to adapt and adopt new strategies, Jonathan Sadowsky's closing essay reminds us of a crucial element of continuity – the legacies of colonialism. The emphasis on colonialism may impart too much weight to the role of the state, and underestimate African agency, but without taking into account the persistent physical, socio-structural and epistemological colonial shadows, it is difficult to understand illness and healthcare in Africa, he argues. Pervading the varied, multidisciplinary studies in this volume, lies what Sadowsky calls an "epistemological violence." Its persistent reality, often neglected by scholars and the public, is one of the main reasons why we study medicine in Africa.

Notes

[1]See, e.g.: Tracy J. Luedke and Harry G. West, eds., *Borders and Healers: Brokering Therapeutic Resources in Southeast Africa* (Bloomington: Indiana University Press, 2006); Credo Vusa'mazulu Mutwa, *Zulu Shaman: Dreams, Prophecies, and Mysteries* (Rochester, VT: Destiny Books, 2003); Edward Green, *Aids and STDs in Africa: Bridging the Gap between Traditional Healing and Modern Medicine* (Boulder, CO: Westview Press, 1994); Edward C. Green, *Indigenous Theories of Contagious Disease* (Walnut Creek, CA.: AltaMira Press, 1999); Isaac Sindiga et al., eds., *Traditional Medicine in Africa* (Nairobi: East African Educational Publishers, 1995); Gloria M. Waite, *A History of Traditional Medicine and Health Care in Pre-colonial East-Central Africa* (Lewiston, NY: E. Mellen Press, 1992); Ngoma John Janzen, *Discourses of Healing in Central and Southern Africa* (Berkeley: University of California Press, 1992); John Gray, *Àshe, Traditional Religion and Healing in Sub-Saharan Africa and the Diaspora: A Classified International Bibliography* (New York: Greenwood Press, 1989); John Gray, Anita Jacobson-Widding and David Westerlund, eds., *Culture, Experience and Pluralism: Essays on African Ideas of Illness and Healing* (Uppsala: Academiae Upsaliensis, 1989); Akin M. Makinde, *African Philosophy, Culture, and Traditional Medicine* (Athens, Ohio: Ohio University Press, 1988).

[2]See, e.g.: Jean-Paul Bado, ed., *Les conquêtes de la médecine moderne en Afrique* (Paris: Karthala, 2006); André Audoynaud, *Le docteur Schweitzer et son hospital à Lambaréné: l'envers d'un mythe* (Paris: L'Harmattan, 2005); Colin Murray and Peter Sanders, *Medicine Murder in Colonial Lesotho: The Anatomy of a Moral Crisis* (Edinburgh: Edinburgh University Press, 2005); Kirk Arden Hoppe, *Lords of the Fly: Sleeping Sickness Control in British East Africa, 1900-1960* (Westport, CT: Praeger, 2003); Cynthia Brantley, *Feeding Families: African Realities and British Ideas of Nutrition and Development in Early Colonial Africa* (Portsmouth, NH: Heinneman, 2002); Myron Echenberg, *Black Death, White Medicine: Bubonic Plague and the Politics of Public Health in Colonial Senegal* (Portsmouth, NH: Heinemann, 2002); Osaak A. Olumwullah, *Disease in the Colonial State: Medicine, Society and Social Change among the Abanyole of Western Kenya* (Westport, CT: Greenwood Press, 2002); Diana Wylie, *Starving on a Full Stomach: Hunger and the Triumph of Cultural Racism in Modern South Africa* (Charlottesville: University Press of Virginia, 2001); Roy MacLeod, ed., *Nature and Empire: Science and the Colonial Enterprise* (Osiris, 2nd series, 15, Chicago: University of Chicago Press, 2000); Jonathan Sadowsky, *Imperial Bedlam: Institutions of Madness in Colonial Southwest Nigeria* (Berkeley: University of California Press, 1999); E. Sylla, *'People Are not the Same': Leprosy and Identity in the Twentieth Century Mali* (Portsmouth, NH: Heinemann, 1998); Jean-Paul Bado, *Médecine coloniale et grandes endémies en Afrique 1900-1960 : Lèpre, trypanosomiase et onchocercose* (Paris:

Karthala, 2003); Dagmar Engels and Shula Marks, eds., *Contesting Colonial Hegemony: State and Society in Africa and India* (New York: I.B. Tauris, 1994); Steven Feierman and John M. Janzen, eds., *The Social Basis of Health and Healing in Africa* (Berkeley: University of California Press, 1992); Maryinez Lyons, *The Colonial Disease: A Social History of Sleeping Sickness in Northern Zaire, 1900-1940* (New York: Cambridge University Press, 1992, 2002); John Farley, *Bilharzia: A History of Imperial Tropical Medicine* (New York: Cambridge University Press, 1991); N.E. Gallagher, *Egypt's Other Wars: Epidemics and the Politics of Public Health* (Syracuse, NY: University of Syracuse Press, 1990); Philip Curtin, *Death by Migration: Europe's Encounter with the Tropical World in the Nineteenth Century* (New York: Cambridge University Press, 1989); Randall Packard, *White Plague, Black Labor: Tuberculosis and the Political Economy of Health and Disease in South Africa* (Berkeley: University of California Press, 1989); Roy MacLeod and Milton Lewis, eds., *Disease, Medicine, and Empire: Perspectives on Western Medicine and the Experience of European Expansion* (London: Routledge, 1988).

[3]See, e.g.: Lynn M. Thomas, *Politics of the Womb: Women, Reproduction, and the State in Kenya* (Berkeley: University of California Press, 2003); Diana Wylie, *Starving on a Full Stomach: Hunger and the Triumph of Cultural Racism in Modern South Africa* (Charlottesville: University Press of Virginia, 2001); Alan Bewell, *Romanticism and Colonial Disease* (Baltimore: Johns Hopkins University Press, 1999); Nancy R. Hunt, *A Colonial Lexicon of Birth Ritual, Medicalization, and Mobility in the Congo* (Durham, NC: Duke University Press, 1999); Philip W. Setel et al., *Histories of Sexually Transmitted Disease and HIV/AIDS in Sub-Saharan Africa* (Westport, CT.: Greenwood Press, 1999); Meredeth Turshen, *Privatizing Health Services in Africa* (New Brunswick: Rutgers University Press, 1999); Teresa Meade and Mark Walker, eds., *Science, Medicine, and Cultural Imperialism* (New York: St. Martin's Press, 1991).

[4]John Iliffe, *East African Doctors: A History of the Modern Profession* (New York: Cambridge University Press, 1998); Adell Patton, Physicians, *Colonial Racism, and Diaspora in West Africa* (Gainesville: University Press of Florida, 1996); Murray Last and G.L. Chavunduka, eds., *The Professionalisation of African Medicine* (Manchester: Manchester University Press, 1986).

[5]Eilleen Stillwaggon, *AIDS and the Ecology of Poverty* (London: Oxford University Press, 2006); Nana K. Poku, *AIDS in Africa. How the Poor are Dying* (Cambridge, UK: Polity Press, 2005); Alexander Irwin et al., *Global AIDS: Myths and Facts. Tools for Fighting the AIDS Pandemic* (Cambridge, MA: South End Press, 2004); Max Essex et al., *AIDS in Africa* (New York: Kluwer Academic/Plenum Publishers, 2002); Edward Green, *AIDS and STDs in Africa: Bridging the Gap between Traditional Healing and Modern Medicine* (Boulder, CO: Westview Press, 1994).

[6]Frank Ham, *AIDS in Africa: How Did It Ever Happen?* (Zomba, Malawi: Kachere Series, 2004); Michelle Cochrane, *When AIDS Began: San Francisco and the Making of an Epidemic* (New York: Routledge, 2004); Cindy Patton, *Inventing AIDS* (New York: Routledge, 1990).

[7]Alex Preda, *AIDS, Rhetoric, and Medical Knowledge* (New York: Cambridge University Press, 2005); Edward Green, *Rethinking AIDS Prevention: Learning from Successes in Developing Countries* (Wesport, CT.: Praeger, 2003).

[8] Elizabeth Fee and Daniel M. Fox, eds., *AIDS: The Burdens of History* (Berkeley: University of California Press, 1989); Norman Miller and Richard Rockwell, eds., *AIDS*

in Africa: The Social and Policy Impact (New York: The Edwin Mellon Press, 1988).

[9]Michelle Cochrane, *When AIDS Began*, xxiii.

[10]Philip D. Curtin, "The White Man's Grave: Image and Reality, 1780-1850," *Journal of British Studies*, 1 (1961): 94-110; Philip D. Curtin, "The End of the 'White Man's Grave'? Nineteenth-Century Mortality in West Africa," *Journal of Interdisciplinary History*, 21 (1990): 63-88.

[11]Kalala Ngalamulume, "Keeping the City Totally Clean: Yellow Fever and the Politics of Prevention in Colonial Saint-Louis du Sénégal, 1850-1914," *Journal of African History*, 45 (2004): 183-202.

[12]Paula A. Treichler, *How to Have Theory in an Epidemic: Cultural Chronicles of AIDS* (Durham: Duke University Press, 1999).

[13]Oppong and Jayati Ghosh, "Concluding Remarks: Beyond Epidemiology," in *HIV and AIDS in Africa, Beyond Epidemiology*, ed. Ezekiel Kalipeni et al. (Malden, MA: Blackwell Publishing, 2004), 323-4.

[14]Charles E. Rosenberg, Introduction to *Framing Disease. Studies in Cultural History*, ed. Charles E. Rosenberg and Janet Golden (New Brunswick, NJ: Rutgers University Press, 1992), xviii.

[15]Jean Comaroff, *Body of Power, Spirit of Resistance: The Culture and History of a South African People* (Chicago: The University of Chicago Press, 1985).

[16]S. Leonard Syme and Lisa F. Berkman, "Social Class, Susceptibility, and Sickness," in *The Sociology of Health and Illness: Critical Perspective*, ed. Peter Conrad and Rochelle Kern (New York: St. Martin's Press, 1986), 29-30; Steven Feierman and JohnM. Janzen, eds., *The Social Basis of Health and Healing in Africa* (Berkeley: University of California Press, 1992), 8.

[17]Kalipeni et al., eds., *HIV and AIDS in Africa*. For the negative images of Africa, see also Jean and John Comaroff, *Ethnography and the Historical Imagination* (Boulder, CO: Westview Press, 1992), 215-233.

[18]Lawrence Adeokun, "Social and Cultural Factors Affecting the HIV Epidemic," in *AIDS in Nigeria: A Nation on the Threshold*, ed. Olusoji Adeyi et al. (Cambridge, MA: Harvard Center for Population and Development Studies, 2006), 151-173.

[19]Cindy Patton, *Inventing AIDS* (New York: Routledge, 1990), 77, 82, 86-7.

[20]Emiko Ohnuki-Thierney, ed., *Culture through Time: Anthropological Approaches* (Stanford: Stanford University Press, 1990).

[21]Margaret Humphreys, "Kicking a Dying Dog: DDT and the Demise of Malaria in the American South, 1942-1950," *Isis*, 87 (1996): 2.

[22]David N. Nabarro and Elizabeth M. Tayler, "The 'Roll Back Malaria' Campaign," *Science*, 280 (1998): 2067.

[23]Richard A. Liroff, "DDT Risk Assessments: Response," *Environmental Health Perspectives*, 109 (2001): A302.

[24]Louis H. Miller, "The Challenge of Malaria," *Science*, 257 (1992): 36.

CHAPTER 2

Is Culture Risky? Media Representations and Local Interpretations of Risk in Western Kenya

CRYSTAL BIRUK

The rate of HIV prevalence in Nyanza Province (15 percent) is more than twice the Kenyan national average of 6 percent, and prevalence among the sub-population of widows may reach 30 percent.[1] The Luo, the largest ethnic group in this province, represented 32.8 percent of the national caseloads in 2000, but comprised only 13 percent of the Kenyan population.[2] Why is prevalence drastically higher among Luo widows? This question has been at the root of HIV education, prevention and public health interventions in this region. The manner in which this question has been answered will form the basis of this paper. I explore the way in which assumptions about risk and meta-discourses[3] about cultural practices in national and international media may inform and dominate discussions about appropriate action and public health interventions to stop the spread of HIV/AIDS. In Kenya, national and international media frequently place the blame for Nyanza's HIV problem on the traditional Luo practice of widow inheritance, or *ter*. This practice involves the inheritance of a widow by her deceased husband's brother-in-law or some other male kin.[4]

The grim statistics that come in the wake of the HIV/AIDS epidemic in sub-Saharan Africa have prompted a scrutinizing of acts previously construed as private or under the umbrella of individual rights, in the name of public health and AIDS prevention. In sub-Saharan Africa, sexual and cultural practices in areas of high HIV prevalence (e.g. sexual cleansing, female circumcision, polygamy) have been represented as dangerous, primitive and unhealthy. This paper uses widow inheritance in western Kenya as a specific example of the discordance between 1) the discursive object[5] of widow inheritance created through media representation and 2) the way in which local actors engaged in these practices may perceive the tradition and its association with HIV/AIDS risk. My paper draws on three months of research in western Kenya in the Summer of 2004. My thinking about this issue was further influenced by two months spent in rural Malawi in 2005.

Methods

This paper is based on content analysis of newspaper stories about cultural practices and HIV/AIDS from the time period 1997-2005. Articles were collected during my time in Kenya and Malawi (Summers of 2002, 2004 and 2005) and through online archive searches of newspaper sources. Relevant articles were coded using the software package NUD*IST,[6] with special attention paid to the types of adjectives used to refer to cultural practices. The paper also draws on 40 semi-structured interviews I conducted with widows from Nyanza Province, aged 18-49.[7] Most of the women I talked with were between 30 and 44 years of age and had attended primary school. Women primarily worked as small-scale farmers, small-scale business women, or just found work as it was available. Finally, the overwhelming majority of the women I spoke with made less than 1000 Kenya shillings per month (at the time, about USD 12.50). In addition to conducting the interviews, I got a sense of the cultural environment by hanging around the health clinic, chatting with women whenever I was able to, playing with their children, and shopping in the market. Women were generally happy to speak with me; they seemed excited to share their comments on widow inheritance and "being Luo" with me.

Media representations of Luo cultural practices

In general, the media represents *ter* as the main cause for elevated HIV rates in western Kenya. The Kenyan daily newspaper *The Nation* often features discussions and debates about the high HIV/AIDS prevalence within the country. Frequently, this discourse works to localize or containerize AIDS to western Kenya, relegating the epidemic to a specific region, ethnic group, and set of cultural practices. As the Luo are already set off from the rest of the country politically, economically and culturally, these representations likely reinvigorate popular stereotypes of this part of the country. Here,

I list some headlines concerning widow inheritance and other "dangerous traditions" that appeared relatively recently in both international and national media sources. The headlines come from a variety of sources ranging from well-known international newspapers to local African newspapers:

"Kenyan Widows' New **Fear**: Many women in the East African nation are 'inherited' by male in-laws who marry them after their husbands die. Opponents of the **ancient custom** say it's fostering the spread of AIDS" (*Los Angeles Times*, 1998)

"**Justice** for **Vulnerable** Widows in Uganda" (Christian Reformed World Relief Committee, 2002)

"Wife Inheritance **Spurs AIDS Rise** in Kenya" (*Washington Post*, 1997)

"Rights group **calls for an end** to inheriting African widows" (*New York Times*, 2003)

"**Tackling** the Impact of Customs on AIDS" (UN-OCHA Integrated Regional Information Network, 2004)

"**Clash Between Tradition and Common Sense**" (*The Nation*, 2004)

"Tanzanian castrates self **in protest** over widow inheritance" (*East African Standard*, 2004)

"Ban **explicit** dances" (*The Malawi Times*, 2005)

"AIDS Now Compels Africa to **Challenge Widows' Cleansing**" (*New York Times*, 2005)

"Bakiga **warned** on wife inheritance" (*The Guardian*, 2004)

Note the words used above. They often carry with them great affect, generating a series of thoughts and images that serve to naturalize and legitimate the idea that traditions may be inimical to health or humanitarian concerns. They also serve to bring into the reader's imagination particular kinds of subjects that become moralized through certain cultural practices that may be deemed good or bad, healthy or unhealthy. The anthropologist

Henrietta Moore writes that "The text takes as its object – its subject for representation – not the 'real' but certain significations and representations about the real."[8] So, when distant (or local) readers hear about dangerous and risky cultural practices killing helpless and passive Africans, it is clear that this imaginary is only one of many, and that representation always only glosses the complexity of the actual situation. Susan Sontag's observation that "the Other ... is someone to be seen, not someone (like us) who also sees"[9] indexes the manner in which the representational field[10] is controlled by those who have a monopoly on representation and interpretation. Those people and institutions who are doing what Sontag refers to as "the seeing" determine which images and discourses percolate the public sphere, while those who are "seen" are often glossed and divested of agency and voice by these textual representations.

The bulk of articles I surveyed portray inheritance and other practices as ancient customs out of place in a fast-paced globalized world. Many of these articles also utilize human rights jargon (that is, words like "justice," "calls for an end," "in protest") which builds on the legitimacy garnered by the framing of HIV/AIDS as a public health issue. Blaming widow inheritance for high HIV prevalence in Nyanza is justified first, because it is a threat to public health and second, because of the threat it poses to human and women's rights. Finally, words like "warned" and "tackling" invoke a number of dichotomies: science/tradition, state/ethnic group, and rational/irrational.

These representations point to the tendency to blame failed public health interventions or development agendas on African customs and resistance to change. In fact, public health documents often incorporate these very same discourses and representations. For example, the 2001 Balaka District Plan for HIV/AIDS, in a rural sector of Malawi, states that one of the main areas of focus is "the culture which promotes the spread of HIV/AIDS," and names traditional authorities as "agents of development" who will filter messages to their publics. The 2002 Kenyan AIDS Control Council Sub-committee on Gender Report lists cultural practices like inheritance and circumcision as cultural contributors to what it terms "gender vulnerability factors."[11] Similarly, the World Health Organization (WHO) lists "harmful cultural practices" as one of its main areas of focus for public health (particularly women's health) improvement in sub-Saharan Africa.[12] By virtue of geographical distance from the setting of these maligned cultural practices, audiences may accept as fact the representations crafted by the media and other sources. Representations of HIV/AIDS in Africa also reinvigorate a set of familiar stereotypes leading to the interpretation of the AIDS "plague" as a judgment on a society that is entrenched in backwardness and shackled to tradition. Machungo terms this emphasis on cultural and traditional precursors to AIDS as the "cultural fixation" of the U.S. media, which places almost exclusive attention on cultural-related, so-called risky behaviors, as opposed to other factors.[13]

The demonization of cultural practices in diverse sources indicates that cultural practices are the *only* possible cause for the elevated rates of HIV in local regions, and the dire impact of HIV/AIDS on public health justify this conclusion. In western Kenya, for example, widow inheritance is represented as dangerous, risky and unhealthy. However, other sources may tell a different story. For example, the way that local Luo women talk about widow inheritance indicates that the picture provided by media and other accounts is incomplete and may not effectively represent the experience of all women, or even of the average woman. In brief interviews with forty Luo widows, I noted that local perceptions and assessments of HIV/AIDS risk may differ drastically from dominant representations. I hypothesize that women's discussions of HIV/AIDS and *ter* are impacted by globalized discourses that circulate in Nyanza, but that their stance on widow inheritance and how risky they view it to be are by no means aligned with international representations of their experience and supposed vulnerability. I suggest that incorporating local narratives and perceptions of risk into public health planning and interventions may result in better health outcomes. In the next section, I overview the main themes that colored my conversations with Luo widows about widow inheritance and AIDS.

The Way Things Were: "In the Old Days..."

A theme that ran through almost all of the interviews was the blurring of boundaries that, not long ago, used to be visible and well-demarcated in certain ways. Women talked about how there is little observable difference between mothers and daughters, or ladies and young girls. Many of their statements implied an erosion of cultural rules and social regulations on female behavior. This general view of Luo women, especially young women, as free or unconstrained may have implications for women's beliefs about the spread of HIV/AIDS. Specifically, women talked about Luo tradition and culture as a "container" that could be protective against female promiscuity. For example, a woman is often referred to as "free" if she is not inherited following the death of her brother-in-law. Though this might index certain positive notions of female empowerment, in Luoland a free woman can be viewed as promiscuous or improper. This seems to contradict the humanitarian agenda of freeing Luo women from widow inheritance and empowering women to resist inheritance. If local women associate tradition with a protective effect against immorality and promiscuity (and thus, by extension, HIV/AIDS transmission), then efforts to change this practice are likely to be confounded and ineffective.

"She Moves a Lot": Insider/Outsider Notions of Risk

Though almost all women in my sample described widow inheritance or inheritors as "risky" or "dangerous" and recognized that it "spreads disease," it is essential to recognize the very specific aspects of inheritance practice that are associated with risk and disease. Women do not view widow inheritance monolithically as "risky," but instead pointed to certain aspects of its practice that they deem risky. Respondents in Agot's study cited a number of recent changes in the practice of widow inheritance. The main change was the increase in professional inheritors, or men who pass through town inheriting women and attaining associated benefits for the time they are with them. Because these men are doing the woman and her family a favor by facilitating her *chodo* or cleansing,[14] they may feel entitled to good food, shelter and sex.[15] Similarly, my interviews indicated that these professional inheritors move all around Nyanza province looking for women to inherit; in fact, women often claimed that many professional inheritors were not even Luo, but traveled from other parts of Kenya or Uganda.

Though most of the widows I spoke with referred to "risk" or "disease" in discussions of widow inheritance, these terms only mapped directly onto things, people and concepts deemed to be "outside," or "foreign" to Luo culture. First, women often discussed professional inheritors in this manner, referring to their roots outside the local community, the risk from "outside" or the lack of "background checks" on professional inheritors. They associated risk and susceptibility to HIV with professional inheritors, whom they view as "brokers of disease." Because these men are not from the local community, it is impossible for either the widow or her family to know their background (sexual and other). Thus, the professional inheritor, *but not necessarily inheritance itself*, has come to symbolize risk, danger and the unknown.

Urban Risk

The salience of the insider/outsider construct for risk is also noted in discussions of location, and the association of disease with other "foreign" invasions such as Western-influenced moralities. In the interviews, there was a strong association between urban areas and disease. Women spoke of widows looking for another partner in a "different town." They also associated urban areas with spending "less time with grandparents" and blamed this on the influence of Western culture. Many told me about women who moved away temporarily to towns or cities and came back infected with HIV/AIDS. The polarization of urban and rural mirrors the associations of risk and immorality with places "outside" the local. Women search for men in "different towns" or move to urban areas and, it is implied, bring back HIV/AIDS. Thus, threats to health are located in places that are distant to the immediate environment of Luo women.

Women also located risk in or as stemming from "Western culture." In many cases, the "Western" is contrasted with "the Luo." Although the presence of Westerners and Western culture may primarily be a response to the extraordinarily high rates of HIV prevalence in Nyanza, Luo widows view Western culture as essentially opposed to, or at war with traditional culture ("traditional culture is being outlawed by Western culture" and "Western culture may have an upper hand"). Women recognized that their local context is becoming more urbanized due to the influx of people and funding associated with large-scale public health projects targeting HIV and widow inheritance behavior change. Ironically, it is in these health workers and their novelty that women see "risk." For example, women told me about how men come from all over Kenya to work in their province, and often end up having sexual relations with some of the women in Nyanza. They associate Western culture with moral degeneration, exposure to new value systems, promiscuity, and inappropriate sexual behavior.

"Movement"

Many widows utilized the verb "to move" to refer to promiscuous, irresponsible and immoral sexual behavior, and prostitution among women. For the most part, it appeared tightly linked to expressions of female promiscuity. Some examples include talk of young ladies moving for large sums of money, girls who come from irresponsible families moving a lot, and women being unsettled, or "walking up and down." The association of the verb "to move" with promiscuity and immorality is telling, in light of the insider/outsider risk construct, and the notion of Luo identity and widow inheritance itself as protective against the foreign invasions of HIV and Western culture. Specifically, women who "move" are transgressing important boundaries that have only recently become malleable. Thus, although widows express a certain amount of disdain for the practice of inheritance, they appreciate its ability to "contain" women who would otherwise "move" around and spread disease. The use of the verb "to move" also surfaced in discussions of female promiscuity in Malawi, where locals have even adopted an adjective that incorporates this verb – *movious*.

Conclusions

Though this paper only begins to address much larger issues that should be studied further, it is clear that representations of HIV/AIDS risk as rooted in cultural practices should be interrogated. Indeed, the conflation of human rights and public health discourses inherently justifies and legitimates the idea of cultural practice as risky. It is clear that local perceptions of risk should be incorporated into interventions for HIV/AIDS, as they may problematize the dominant epidemiological and biomedical focus on certain practices as threatening to public health. The "cultural fixation"[16] of the media facilitates a myopia that normalizes and corroborates the logic of blaming AIDS on culture, backwardness and tradition. The late Susan Sontag suggests that a situation must be transformed into a spectacle to become interesting to its audiences. It is important to acknowledge the primary role played by the "representational field" in determining *which* representations percolate in the media. As this small study has shown, the media "object" of widow inheritance only begins to gloss the nuances and complexities of the actual practice of the tradition. Of course, the stories told by local women are also only representations. Like the media, these representations are constrained by the mode, audience (me, an anthropologist) and context. For example, although most of the women told me widow inheritance used to be practiced differently, it would be silly to assume that it has an original form, or that the stories these women told me were not informed by nostalgia and awareness that I knew little about widow inheritance. However, in seeking representations from various sources, including local actors, I think a more nuanced version of the elusive "truth" may be achieved.

This paper juxtaposes media and local interpretations of risk and cultural practice. Its call to challenge monolithic, linear, and biomedical notions of risk or health comes out of critical medical anthropology.[17] In this tradition, the paper suggests that we should interrogate dominant views of risk even if they are corroborated by a benevolent concern with the public's health. It also points to the way in which certain human behaviors and groups of people are moralized and marked in the face of high prevalence of or elevated concern about HIV/AIDS.[18] Paul Rabinow suggests that human rights might be the most powerful and least challengeable discourse that moves through the world.[19] The discipline of public health, too, enjoys a certain authority that stems from its legitimate ability to regulate human behavior in the name of the public good. However, the authoritative power of these discourses should not cloud our ability to critically assess assumptions and intentions around complicated concepts like risk, culture and HIV/AIDS in Africa. Further research in this area will destabilize biomedical notions of risk, facilitate critical reflexivity in thinking about HIV/AIDS risk in sub-Saharan Africa, and challenge the assumptions that authoritative "speakers" in biomedical, public health and human rights institutions make about the HIV/AIDS epidemic and cultural practice. Additionally, and importantly, it will complement outside analyses of cultural practice with local assessments and descriptions of the behavior under question.

Acknowledgements

The author would like to thank the following: Dr. Kawango Agot, Onyango Mathews, UNIM Project (Kisumu, Kenya), HAWI Project (Bondo, Kenya), the Fogarty International Center, NIH #1 R01 TW06230-01. Her experience with the Malawi Diffusion and Ideational Change Project (MDICP) and Malawi Religion Project (MRP) were also instrumental in forming her thinking about these issues.

Notes

[1] A. R. Cross et al, "Sociodemographic and Behavioral Correlates of HIV Prevalence in Kenya" (paper presented at the Fifteenth International Conference on AIDS, Bangkok, Thailand, July 11-16, 2004).

[2] Kawango Agot, "Widow Inheritance and HIV/AIDS Interventions in Sub-Saharan Africa: Contrasting Conceptualizations of 'Risk' and 'Spaces of Vulnerability'" (PhD diss, University of Washington, 2001).

[3] The term meta-discourses refers here to talk about talk, or commentary on commentary. See Greg Urban, *Meta-Culture: How Culture Moves Through the World* (Minneapolis: University of Minnesota Press, 2001).

[4] See Agot, "Widow Inheritance," 193; Nancy Luke, "Local Meanings and Census Categories: Widow Inheritance and the Position of Luo Widows in Kenya," in *African Households*, ed. Etienne Vande Walle (Armonk, NY: ME Sharpe, Inc., 2005); Isaac Luginaah et al, "Challenges of a Pandemic: HIV/AIDS Related Problems Affecting Kenyan Widows," *Social Science and Medicine* 60 (2005): 1219-1228; Betty Potash, *Widows in African Societies: Choices and Constraints* (Stanford: Stanford University Press, 1986); Wakana Shino, "Widow's Practice of Pro-husband Choice in a Rural Luo Community," *Journal of African Studies* 59 (2001): 71-84.

[5] I use the term "discursive object" to refer to the way that a massive number of representations of widow inheritance and cultural practice in the media have led to the "solidification" over time of a particular imagined object of widow inheritance and cultural practice.

[6] See http://www.qsrinternational.com/

[7] These interviews were conducted in a back room at a rural clinic where we enjoyed privacy. I had an interpreter. I do speak Swahili, so in cases where women spoke Swahili as well as Luo, I used the opportunity to probe and discuss more deeply.

[8] Henrietta L Moore, *Space, Text and Gender: An Anthropological Study of the Marakwet of Kenya* (New York: Guilford Publications, 1996), 94.

[9] Susan Sontag, *Regarding the Pain of Others* (New York: Farrar, Strauss and Giroux, 2003), 72.

[10] Judith Butler, *Precarious Life: The Powers of Mourning and Violence* (New York: Verso, 2004).

[11] See page 13 of the online document: http://www.nacc.or.ke/

[12] See: http://www.who.int/mediacentre/factsheets/fs247/en/

[13] Francis Gatua Machungo, "The Representation of the AIDS Epidemic in Africa by the U.S. Media: A Critical Analysis" (MA thesis, University of Illinois at Urbana-Champaign, 2005), 10-11.

[14] This refers to the sexual cleansing a woman undergoes following the death of her husband. If a family has a difficult time finding a brother in law or other male kin to do the cleansing (often due to belief that the woman may be infected with AIDS), they may hire a professional inheritor.

[15] Agot, "Widow Inheritance," 196.

[16] Machungo, "The Representation of the AIDS Epidemic in Africa."

[17] Linda M. Hunt and Cheryl Mattingly, "Diverse Rationalities and Multiple Realities in Illness and Healing," *Medical Anthropology Quarterly* 12 (1998): 267-72; Arthur Kleinman and Byron Good, *Culture and Depression: Studies in the Anthropology and Cross-Cultural Psychiatry of Affect and Disorder* (Berkeley: University of California Press, 1985); Emily Martin, *The Woman in the Body: A Cultural Analysis of Reproduction* (Boston: Beacon Press, 1987); Lynn Payer, *Medicine and Culture: Varieties of Treatment in the United States, England, West Germany and France* (New York: Henry Holt and Company, 1996); and Nancy Scheper-Hughes and Margaret Lock, "The Mindful Body: A Prolegomenon to Future Work in Medical Anthropology," In *Understanding and Applying Medical Anthropology*, ed. Peter J. Brown (Mountain View, CA: Mayfield Publishing Company, 1998).

[18] Douglas Crimp, *Melancholia and Moralism: Essays on AIDS and Queer Politics* (Boston: MIT Press, 2002); Paul Farmer, *AIDS and Accusation: Haiti and the Geography of Blame* (Berkeley: University of California Press, 1992).

[19] Paul Rabinow, *Anthropos Today: Reflections on Modern Equipment* (Princeton: Princeton University Press, 2003).

Chapter 3

The Politics of HIV Education for Adolescents in South Africa

Zolani Ngwane

Introduction

In South Africa over 5 million people are living with HIV, the largest number in the world.[1] Young people between ages of 15 and 25 are the most vulnerable to the disease, particularly females.[2] The principal mode of transmission in South Africa is unprotected sex between a male and a female. Studies have identified a number of mediating factors for such high rates of infection, including the attenuated initial response by the government;[3] poverty;[4] unemployment and migration;[5] and escalating cases of violent sexual assault, particularly on women and children.[6]

As hopes for a quick medical solution to the pandemic began to fade, research and advocacy turned to prevention as the most effective strategy. The method widely used involved educating the public about the disease, which took the form of disseminating information through radio, television, newspaper inserts, pamphlets, public theatrical performances, billboards, etc. Public schools upgraded their Life Skills curriculum to include information about HIV/AIDS. This mass circulation of knowledge had the advantage of reaching large numbers of people simultaneously, thus reducing costs. The assumption behind this approach was that correct knowledge would enable people to make the right choices to protect themselves.

It soon became clear, however, that knowledge by itself was not enough to arrest the spread of the disease, and that in addition to this approach interventions targeting the modification of behavior and providing practical skills would be necessary.[7] Research soon indicated that besides socioeconomic variables such as poverty and unemployment, there were other structural factors that predisposed people to HIV infection. This new set of variables – "cultural norms," "social norms," "shared meanings" – identified certain African cultural practices as HIV risk factors. The following are a few examples:

a) Polygyny, which is no longer widely practiced in South Africa, but whose legacy is argued to still "sanction(s) the principle that African males can have a variety of female sexual partners,"[8] thus undermining the provision for gender equality in the country's constitution;[9]

b) *Lobola* (bridewealth), "a contract between men about a woman,"[10] which reduces a married woman to her husband's "property,"[11] eliminating her ability to negotiate safe sex within marriage, while obligating her to his sexual demands at the pain of violence or rejection;[12]

c) Patriarchy, a form of gerontocracy whose enforcement of respect for elders puts young people, especially females, at risk of sexual exploitation by older men.[13] Patriarchy also promotes child rape through its associated belief that having sex with a virgin helps cure STDs,[14] and it cultivates a culture of "'machismo" among young males, which manifests itself in violence against women and a tendency to have multiple sexual partner;[15]

d) Beliefs, attitudes, views and actions that are rationalized by those who hold them as part of, or as sanctioned by their culture.

This research on cultural mediators of sexual behavior produced important information on the life circumstances of the people most affected by the disease. For example, within the first ten years of its existence, the Gender Research Project of the University of Witwatersrand has courageously shaped public debates on the role of Customary Law in perpetuating gender inequalities (through its provision for polygyny and bridewealth, for example) and in compromising women's ability to negotiate safe sex within marriage. The Working Paper Series of the Centre for Social Science Research at the University of Cape Town has published original research on the cultural context of HIV stigma and safe sex behavior. Individual scholars and Non-Governmental Organizations (NGOs) have also produced reliable statistical data on the correlation between violence against women and children, and the rates of HIV infection.

The output of this body of work will continue to make it possible to design and implement effective interventions, to raise public awareness about ongoing inequalities, and to organize policy initiatives aimed at redressing the legal position of women and children in society. The emphasis on the context of behavior has helped to counter stigmatizing stereotypes of HIV/AIDS victims as inherently irresponsible, ignorant and promiscuous. It has shown that while individuals may have the ability and right to make choices, these choices are always mediated by structural factors such as laws, beliefs or norms, which often invest some categories of people (males, for example) with power and privilege over others. Conclusions drawn from this work have pointed to the need for interventions aimed at empowering women and changing the beliefs and behaviors of men. A few have called for the illegalization of cultural practices such as *lobola*,[16] while others have advocated changing the practice for the benefit of the marrying couple, instead of enriching the bride's parents.

My paper seeks to complement this work by drawing attention to the other side of the coin, one which is often neglected in the literature – a possible reification of the African culture as the problem end of a binary at whose solution end is biomedical discourse. This way of stating the issue may appear to undermine the important studies I have reviewed above through a reverse reification of African culture as a victim of Western prejudice. On the contrary, my interest is to bring the conversation back to the pressing task at hand, which is to encourage preventive behaviors, by pointing to a neglected space between cultural institutions like *lobola*, which mediate risky behaviors, and the rationalization of these behaviors by individuals. That interstitial space refers to the daily, routine things people do (and the ways in which they do them) to keep themselves safe. In other words, between the cultural forces (and their norms) that structure human behavior, and the conscious rationalization of beliefs and attitudes by individuals, lies the amorphous sphere of mundane practices (and their contingent strategies) that make everyday life. It is here that the distinction between cultural and biomedical knowledge collapses, as people use whatever works to respond to their immediate environment. It is this sphere, I argue, that should serve as the starting point for thinking about and planning prevention interventions.

The emphasis on practice, alongside the normative structures and human reason that mediate it, directs attention to another frontier in the fight against HIV/AIDS – the reinforcement of already existing strategies that people employ to make life under the formalities of culture. Both to defend African culture against perceived prejudice and to set it up as a problem have the same effect of overlooking practice. This is not to deny or belittle the force of macro-level mediators, but merely to recognize that these determinants do not exhaustively explain the contingent details of human practices. It is to recognize that women and young people have neither merely survived culture nor false-consciously reproduced it, but have instead found ways, under the very shadow of culture, to do precisely the things that are represented as culturally forbidden. This is also not to underestimate the conviction with which people invoke the category of culture, but merely to caution that, like all abstract categories, culture reveals as much as it hides.

Consider this example from rural Transkei, where both men and women readily assert that cattle are the prerogatives of men, and that women should not go inside the cattle enclosure. In most of this area, however, the long absence of men due to migrant labor has reshaped domestic economy such that, for more than a hundred years, women have been dealing with cattle and moving in circles forbidden to them by cultural norms. Why, then, do people hold on to cultural beliefs even when their empirical bases are no longer in place? Indeed, how can we explain the discrepancy between the things people do and how they sometimes explain those things?

One way of accounting for this is to see culture as a construct which enables people to make rational generalizations about their actions and beliefs. Culture in this abstract sense may make certain actions understandable because of their connection to a common belief, but culture and the beliefs associated with it are not enough to explain each action carried out in their name. For example, many Xhosa speaking young males in the Eastern Cape go through the initiation rite of circumcision as part of a cultural belief that this ritual transforms boys into men. This belief, however, does not explain the fact that rural young males show less enthusiasm towards the ritual (seeing it at most as something they have to do) than their urban counterparts in places like Mdantsane, who view it as an important mark of their identity as males. Since most people tend to view rural areas as more traditional than urban townships, this situation sounds counter-intuitive. To explain it, we would have to go beyond culture itself, and look at those specific characteristics of the urban experience to which young males see the rite of circumcision as an appropriate response. What explains the differences are not the rules of the ritual (both rural and urban people give the same account of how the ritual is properly done), but the manner in which it features as a strategy or resource that reinforces arguments about urban masculinity.

Another way of explaining the discrepancy between the things people do and their cultural accounts for them is that culture gives a sense of order and continuity to the diffuse experiences of social life, giving people a feeling of control over their lives. This is why appeals to culture are usually stronger in moments of social crisis or change. In such times, people may view their troubled present as the result of departure from culture, which may then be sought after as a cure. Culture and the past in this context are simply a way of regaining some control over social relations. The revival of virginity testing for girls in some parts of South Africa as a way of preventing the spread of HIV, by discouraging girls from engaging in pre-marital sex, is a good example.[17] In a patriarchal context described above, where women in general and girls in particular have little power to negotiate sex, it is easy to see that virginity testing will not go far enough. The popularity of the practice may be explained by a variety of current factors, like male anxieties over perceived loss of social and economic power to women in general. Thus the significance of virginity testing goes beyond the utilitarian goal of preventing HIV infections. In this context of uncertainty and anxieties, culture restores a modicum of stability (but not gender equality) to a fractured world.

In the age of HIV/AIDS, and thus in a world even more complexly fractured, culture has emerged as "a well-defined system of expectations," as Beck found out in a study of Xhosa-speaking, male, antiretroviral-treatment recipients in Cape Town. The following are examples of very common claims among younger males in the Eastern Cape: "homosexuality is not our culture," "in our culture men may have many sexual partner because men cannot help themselves," "condom use is not part of our culture," "in our culture a woman who carries condoms is promiscuous." It is more useful to see assertions like these as arguments about, rather than descriptions of culture. Although they are usually cast in the idiom of the past – "but all men believe in the *Sangoma*,[18] because our fathers believed in the *Sangomas*" – they are nonetheless generated by insecurities in the present. It is important to emphasize that these arguments hardly ever take place in a level playfield. Often generated by real or perceived shifts in relations of social domination (which are generally referred to as the normal way), these arguments tend to both recuperate and naturalize these relations. They are power driven and often backed up by violence. One way of making sense of the escalating violence against women is to look at it as the enforcement of some of these arguments.

To those at the receiving end of these arguments – women, homosexuals and girls – culture in the form presented above may indeed appear as a burden, but the task of critical analysis should go further and identify internal aspects of counter-arguments that could be the starting point for change. The research question, in short, is no longer whether culture in the Eastern Cape allows women to tend cattle (it does not have to) but how they in fact do so. In this way we begin to move from culture as a set of rules, to the strategies by which people conduct their daily lives. It is by looking at the mundane activities behind culture that we will be able to appreciate women and young people, not simply as victims of culture, but also as proactive agents. We will also be able to reinforce preventive behaviors from within the culture itself, instead of limiting ourselves to the discourse of human rights. Given the urgency of the HIV/AIDS situation, the human rights status of cultural practices should be examined alongside the practical work of building on manifest capacities.

To sum, the focus of HIV/AIDS research and advocacy on behavior mediated by cultural norms has produced important data that has helped explain the particular vulnerability of women to HIV infections. However, the debates that this work has incited, about the position of women within African culture and the relevance of certain cultural practices in modern times, have tended to overlook the practice aspect of the question – what sort of strategies people use to avoid and negotiate situations that they perceive as dangerous. These strategies show that cultural hegemony is never complete, but that what often passes for culture are nothing more than contingent arguments backed by violence or threat of it. The actual starting point for theorizing empowerment interventions should be those strategies that are revealed when we rephrase the research question to seek out what people do, instead of what they may or may not do. My concern is not to defend cultural norms that reinforce the silencing of women, nor is it to deny the reality of the violence unleashed in their name. What I am arguing is that when people invoke culture, this too has to be explained instead of accepted as an explanation.

To demonstrate my point about the difference between the polished appearance of culture and the fractured reality of life, I will look at one of the important cultural factors in HIV-prevention interventions with adolescents, a reported normative lack of communication between parents and children, particularly about matters related to sex.[19] This is a well-documented problem, which is also cited as an important factor in the socio-cultural epidemiology of HIV in South Africa. I will discuss this problem using results from a small scale ethnographic research carried out in May 2005, which focused on parent communication with their adolescent children in Mdantsane and C-Section, two urban communities outside the city of East London. I use this ethnographic snapshot to highlight the point I have made above, that culture conceived of as a complete system of procedures and prohibitions does not always determine whether or not people will do certain things. In practice, culture may mask what is otherwise an ensemble of imaginative practices, exchanges, and improvisations, by which people find ways to do things that their present demands of them. The differences in parent-children communication patterns in the two cases I will consider are due to a complex set of local factors, such as insecurity and differential availability of normalizing public institutions like churches. It is factors like these, rather than culture, that shape the strategies people use to communicate with their children.

Local Knowledge and the Epidemiology of HIV

Emagalini (Shacks) or C-Section is a population overflow from Duncan Village – one of the oldest black areas in the East London district of the Eastern Cape, South Africa. C-Section is an informal settlement of about 5000 shacks with a population density of 2500 people per hectar and 200 families to a toilet. Residents in this area come from surrounding rural areas of the old Transkei and Ciskei to which they periodically return for rituals and holidays. Children attend schools in Duncan Village and other areas nearby. Most people in the community work in various service jobs in the city, about one mile away. It was well into the 1990s that the biomedical discourse on HIV/AIDS finally reached places like the C-Section. When I first came to the community, in 1993, knowledge about the disease and the types of people at risk of getting it was still generated and circulated mostly through rumor and gossip. As in many other places with a history of oral social networking, rumor and gossip here played the role of moral coercion, in that they targeted for ridicule and indirect public censorship individuals suspected of deviating from what was considered the norm.

It is in this norm-enforcing mode that rumor and gossip make sense of practices, behaviors or states of affairs – particularly unfamiliar ones – by speculating, not only on their foreign point of origin, but also on the moral deficit in the here and now (as embodied by the subject of rumor, for example) that might explain the events in question. As a form, then, rumor has an inbuilt logic of separation and reincorporation. Behaviors are posted on it until they are perceived as having changed, or until they are normalized over time. Because of the moral import of rumor, the fear of being talked about by others is the most commonly reported form in which people experience stigma. Although it usually takes place in face-to-face encounters in small groups, rumor is a public discourse, which circulates from group to group throughout the community. Following this pattern, information about HIV/AIDS that circulated in the community in the 1990s consisted in various, morally-charged, speculative interpretations of what people had heard from others as well as from the media. In most accounts, HIV was depicted as somewhere else, Port Elizabeth being the most cited place. This location is interesting, because Port Elizabeth is also associated with prevalence and tolerance of homosexuality by many people in the area.[20]

Unlike other diseases, such as tuberculosis, HIV was depicted as a punitive affliction. Within this generally shared moral framework, people had very different views about the moral status of infected individuals once the disease became visible in the area. Among those who believed that witchcraft caused HIV, some were more tolerant of those infected with it, regarding them as victims. Others, however, maintained that the kind of witchcraft which caused HIV was *mphibekelo* (trap), which only works in cases where the intended victim has extra marital affair. One never gets *ibekelo* from a primary relationship, and it is for this reason that HIV-positive people are not regarded as victims, but held responsible for what happen to them. Unfortunately, people in this category tend to regard each infection as if it were primary, lumping together a cheating husband and a wife who gets it from him. A few older women argued that HIV was introduced in the area as a weapon during the political unrests of 1985, and that only over time did it become transmissible by sex and other bodily fluids. All of these different positions were held together by a loose thread of moral discourse, which represented HIV as a violation that was either deserved or maliciously inflicted on the victim. This is important to keep in mind when we talk about norms. This community is made up of people from different areas of the Transkei whose common beliefs may have important differences in details.

HIV knowledge advocacy started relatively late in South Africa in general, and the urgency to disseminate correct information to as many people as possible left no time to try to embed it within already existing local idioms about epidemics, illness and caring for sick people. As a result, HIV/AIDS became abstracted from socially recognizable forms of illness, and instead took the form of a mysterious and foreign disease. When epidemiological details started coming into C-Section from the city via pamphlets people were bringing home, via school children, through radio and television campaigns that were beginning to intensify by the middle of the 1990s, and by word of mouth from the local clinic, it was like a belated signifier that finally found its long lost moral referent. It became the proper name for a preexisting set of moral discourses. In 2002 no one I talked to still referred to HIV as *le nto yase Bhayi* (this thing of Port Elizabeth). It was either called HIV or *le nto ikhoyo* (the thing around). Increase in epidemiological knowledge brought the disease closer.

The association of HIV transmission with bodily fluids fanned people's fears. For most people, blood, semen and breast milk are principles of life and death at the same time. They are essential in the regeneration of life, but they also expose the interiority of the body to outside malignant forces by their tendency to leak. People policed themselves not only against contact with suspected carriers, but also against signs that might betray them as HIV-positive to the rumor circuit. Getting thinner, visiting a clinic, taking any medication, or walking with a limp could mean one had HIV.

Thus, the epidemiological discourse, instead of being a corrective on the cultural myths embodied in the rumors that preceded it, complemented those rumors by making the disease appear peculiar. Where sick people used to be part of public conversations – remembered to neighbors and mentioned in public gatherings like church – the arrival of AIDS discourse resulted in premature social death of many, as families chose silence to exposing themselves to public gossip as victims of the "new thing around." The epidemic soon fitted into the moral categories preceding it, and then coagulated into a discourse of exclusion, difference and distancing. As soon as people knew, thanks to correct epidemiological information, that AIDS did not present in any particularly exotic form of illness, all sick people became available as potential objects of stigma. Stigma here was not the problem of cultural myths resisting scientific truth, but became itself a kind of scientific myth, based on impressively accurate knowledge of the disease's epidemiology.

More relevant to the present discussion, because any individual could already have the disease, HIV/AIDS talk left the sphere of public conversations and receded to the privacy of family homes and close friends. For the most part it found a new public inside the individual household, where parents frequently invoked HIV/AIDS to reign in wayward behavior among children. Each family had rumors about a child in some family who got it either because the parents were too loose or the child too wild. In these home conversations the actual epidemiology of the disease did not really matter. What mattered was the standing of each child within the standards set by the parents. It was the straying outside these standards that put one at risk.

Rules of Language and Strategies of Speech in Parent-Child Communication

Since 2002 I have been a co-investigator in a longitudinal risk-reduction intervention with sixth-grade adolescents in the township of Mdantsane, three miles from C-Section. As a result of my involvement in this study, I became curious about communication between parents and children, particularly about HIV/AIDS. It is a widespread belief that cultural norms prohibit black parents from talking to children about sex-related subjects. My objective was to find out whether, and to what extent, take-home schoolwork had an impact on daily parent-child communication. My long term goal was to find out if school work could be used as an effective strategy in school-based interventions to encourage and regularize conversations about safe behaviors between parents and their children. I looked at two levels of conversation. The first was among parents talking about discussions with their children on various subjects including schoolwork, and the second was between parents and children while the children where doing schoolwork. I randomly selected a group of households to which I had been introduced by friends and colleagues, and had group and individual interviews with parents about their communication patterns with their children. I also sat in to observe the involvement of parents while children were doing their homework.

For the most part, the findings here confirmed what was already generally known, which is that parents feel "culturally unprepared," as one of them put it in a group meeting, to talk to their children about sexually related subjects. They spoke freely about the concerns they had about their children. One parent suspected that her son was smoking, and another said she knew hers was smoking but had not confronted him yet. Parents blamed this to friends with whom they played after school. Concerns about the girls had to do with accidents and forced sex while they run errands for their mothers after school. They also spoke freely about the achievements of their individual children at school and at home. These parents said the same things when I met them in groups and individually. However, their behavior exhibited certain interesting differences when I observed them during the time children were doing homework:

a) While parents in general felt uncomfortable talking to their children about reproductive health, they were more likely to do so if the context was doing school work.

b) When parents were helping the children with their homework a school-type atmosphere was created, the parent assuming an identifiably formal, strict and teacher-like tone. In the course of these homework times the parent could also reproach the child on several other things unrelated to the lesson, such as personal hygiene.

c) Depending on the parent's literacy level, the work would likely be carried out in English, particularly if it involved writing and, more significantly, if the conversation was about sexually related subjects.

In this case, one can see how language use was a key strategy for circumventing what people perceived as a cultural dilemma. Not only was English preferred in talking to children about sex, but the atmosphere itself simulated a school environment. Objectified in this manner, the conversation loses intimacy, and both the interlocutors and the home are distanced from its contents. It is in English and in a simulated classroom. People in general, even in rural areas, seem to think of the school and English language as a morally legitimate medium for communicating sexual material to children. When I asked people whether they thought the church, school or community hall would be the best place to conduct an HIV prevention program, they invariably picked the school. Some explained this choice by pointing out that schools already have posters of anatomical models on their walls.

The roots of this notion that schools and English are the appropriate media for representing material that would not be polite to communicate in Xhosa lie in the 19th century invention of Xhosa as a standard literary language. Alongside the colonial idea that Africans were barbarians, was the assumption that their language needed to be purged before it could become an instrument of civilization. When the missionaries standardized Xhosa as a written language in the 1820s, they took care to substitute descriptive terms for already existing concepts. For example, in the Oxford English Xhosa dictionary, vagina is rendered *indlela eya esizalweni* (a passage to the uterus), a descriptively correct but cumbersome alternative to the more direct concept *inyo*). The resulting standardized Xhosa came to be associated with being Christian and educated, and was distinguished from that spoken by un-converted or "red" Xhosa.[21] Over time the convert/non-convert distinction was replaced by class, so that today polite Xhosa is associated with achievement, success and civilization.

In practice, however, people often face a dilemma when using polite Xhosa, because of its imprecision and sheer wordiness. Even recent dictionaries have resorted to what would earlier have been regarded as vulgar words like *ukudlwengula* – rape – instead of the wordy polite rendition, *ukuzithathela umzimba ongezantsi ngolunya* (to take for oneself the lower body with malice). For the most part, then, people tend to resort to English words in order to be clear, precise and inoffensive. What is interesting is that among themselves most adults freely combine the polite and vulgar Xhosa. With children, however, all sexual references tend to be conveyed in English. I argue that this has become an unconscious strategy to face the reality of having to talk to children about sex-related subjects, while not appearing to contradict what people consider the custom or culture. In the Mdantsane case, therefore, it appeared safe to conclude that school-based prevention interventions should consider incorporating homework assignments that the children can do with their parents, in order to encourage parent-child communication about HIV/AIDS.

It was this possibility that led to my decision to repeat the same study at C-Section, in May 2005. As in Mdantsane, my plan here was to talk to groups of parents, and then spend time with individual families over several evenings to watch interactions between parents and children. Most of the group meetings were held in the home of my host family, who had a relatively bigger space because Mamfene, the mother of the house, was also a traditional healer who often had in-patients staying with the family. Other than the size, the structure of her household was typical of the area. She and her husband, Monde, previously had a rural home about 15 miles away. They moved to C-Section to be with Monde, who worked for the municipality, and to get better schools for their children. Her house was the meeting point for a group of women friends in the community, and this made it easy for me to hold impromptu group interviews.

I had several conversations with mothers of children over four days, and I visited five different families. I worked with a total of nine parents, eight females and one male. Fathers either came home late from work or were otherwise engaged when the children were doing homework. The children were between the ages of 13 and 15. In general, the parents were very knowledgeable about HIV/AIDS, but disagreed about its origins. It was very difficult to get them to talk about their own children in group conversation. They rarely mentioned their children by first names, and used instead generalizing language, like "our children" or "children nowadays." They mentioned school, radio and television as the main sources of knowledge about HIV for children, and most did not think that there was any need for them to talk much to children about the disease. They felt it was more important to teach children to come home straight after school and to help in the house. HIV, like sex and drug use, was a result of indolence and loitering about. When I spoke to these parents individually, in their own homes, they were more willing to talk about their children and their concerns about them specifically. The guarded behavior of parents in C-Section was different from Mdantsane, where parents were very comfortable talking about their own children in public, speaking freely about their bad habits and bragging about good grades and behavior.

In general, parents in Mdantsane created a space for children to do schoolwork and they often helped them. Children were called in from their play to do their homework, and during this time they were either alone in another room or with the parents in the kitchen, if they were working on it together, which happened in most cases. I have already noted the formality with which parents approached this task. By contrast, in C-Section children did homework mostly on their own. Here, because in most cases the room in which children slept was also the family's living and dining rooms, as well as kitchen, all in one, children did their homework in the middle of other house activities. The atmosphere was very informal, parents were often engaged in other things while the children did their homework, and they sometimes even interrupted them if they needed something fetched. In general, the contribution of the parents was minimal. In some of the families they used the time to run errands before it got dark.

In order to understand these differences and to see their implication for parent-child communication, one has to take into consideration the characteristics of the two areas. Mdantsane is a formal township where most of the parents I talked to were born and grew up. A sense of community and continuity is reinforced by historical public institutions and rituals such as churches, schools, weddings, funerals, and local civic and political events. Over time these different institutions have come to mediate a more or less commensurate set of norms that are shared across the community. When norms achieve a level of clarity, people are often free to use innovative strategies in their private pursuit of socially acceptable goals. It is in this private sphere that one can observe improvisations on publicly held norms – some good Christian may also sell marijuana in private. People talk freely about their achievements, but they are not required to disclose how they succeeded. Indeed, a major subject of gossip in Mdantsane was how people made their money. There is an acceptable level of competition for better resources, and people often publicly flaunt their success by extending their houses or buying new cars. This may explain why parents here were more open talking about their individual children in public.

In C-Section, on the other hand, people came from different rural communities, bringing with them slightly different moral lenses for making sense of the world. People's primary cultural allegiance was to these rural communities to which they often returned for weddings, funerals and initiation rites. Because of a lack of space, some people at C-Section held their occasional sacrifices in the homes of relatives in Mdantsane. In a situation like this, norms do not attain a level of clarity and exist merely as loose strands of general agreements about the moral status of certain behaviors. As a result, people feel less safe in public conversations and tend not to disclose details about their private lives. Rumor becomes an ideal normative discourse when it can attribute a problem (HIV) to an outside source (Port Elizabeth). Local people feature as having caught the outside refraction if they are said to behave like, say, people in Port Elizabeth. With the growth of epidemiological knowledge, however, which dismissed the idea of

HIV as something happening elsewhere, people were no longer completely comfortable talking about it in public. HIV left the public level to the more intimate level of family rumor, where it functioned pedagogically, as a way of informing children about behaviors that might lead to HIV infection.

Another important difference between the two communities is the complete lack of public spaces in C-Section. The place is so dense that shacks are only separated by small paths. The shacks themselves are small. The result is a high level of physical intimacy within households. Besides, concerns for security brought kids indoors as soon as it got dark. This means that parents actually spent more time with children here than they did in Mdantsane, and this provided more time for conversation and corrective interventions by parents. Conversations of this sort were scattered through the evening, whereas in Mdantsane they occurred at a particular time. Most of the parents had not gone beyond the fifth grade of school and most families were poorer than those in Mdantsane. This may account for their use of informal Xhosa in front of the children and general openness about sex-related subjects. In this environment, children do their homework in the midst of other regular home activities, and the low literacy may also inhibit parents from active participation in children's schoolwork. Interventions with children in this context may have to adopt a different strategy, which is further complicated by the fact that informal settlements like C-Section do not have their own schools. Children attend schools at nearby townships that may have different characteristics. In this situation, school based interventions may have to be complemented with those targeting parents.

Conclusion

I have talked about two Xhosa-speaking communities where people did not publicly disclose their conversations with children about HIV/AIDS. What accounts for their reluctance to talk about this in public is what they call culture. In the case of Mdantsane I have shown that to understand this culture, one must take into consideration the impact the introduction of Christianity had on Xhosa language and culture in general. In the case of C-Section, the slight differences in cultural understandings of what constitutes appropriate behaviors made people reluctant to divulge intimate information in public. These constraints notwithstanding, I have also shown that in both communities parents in fact do communicate with their children about HIV – mostly in the context of school work in Mdantsane, and in the form of rumor in C-Section. I have argued that the levels at which the conversations take place constitute practical strategies, which often enable people to work around the constraints that culture sometimes imposes on them. The level of strategy, therefore, may be taken to constitute the dynamic element in culture, which also cultivates possible conditions for cultural adaptation or even change. Because our immediate challenge is to encourage behaviors and attitudes that might help reduce people's risk for HIV, we cannot only focus on cultural change, which takes place over a long time and often meets with strong resistance. I have argued that we should instead concentrate our focus on discovering the everyday details of people's practices, within which protective and preventive strategies are often distributed, and make these strategies the main targets of intervention. In the case of Mdantsane, for example, I have suggested that school-based interventions with a well-planned homework component, in which children would be required to work with a parent or caregiver, might be a useful strategy to reinforce parent-child communication. C-Section presents a unique case because a combination of factors such as low literacy and lack of space may make it difficult for parents to be involved in children's homework. Thus, the homework strategy may not apply in all situations.

An important conclusion of this study is that, despite local variations and strategies, parents do communicate with their children about HIV/AIDS. Precisely because of the problems of space both inside and outside individual homes, parents spend more time with their children, giving them the opportunity to talk about HIV/AIDS. The differences between the two cases show that strategies are contingent to social factors, such as availability of public institutions, class, religion and space. These factors are very important to identify in order to be able to get to the strategies that work in a particular environment. All of these different issues, from public assertions about what is culturally appropriate to the private practices that get things done, constitute a complicated politics of HIV education for adolescents in South Africa. They are political because at stake is the organization of social relationships that structure both public and private spheres. Like all politically driven discourse, however, HIV education has its own polished side of shared truths and convictions, as well as an underbelly of competing strategies and unstructured arguments. It is this latter level that I have sought to highlight in this paper as an important starting point for theorizing prevention interventions.

Notes

[1]UNAIDS, *Report on the Global HIV/AIDS Epidemic* (Geneva: World Health Organization, June 2004).

[2]Pretoria Department of Health, "2003 National HIV and Syphillis Antenatal Seroprevalence Survey in South Africa," http://www.dog.gov.za/doc/reports.2002.hivsyphylis; Olive Shisana, and Leickness Simbayi, eds., *Nelson Mandela/HSRC Study of HIV/AIDS: South African National HIV Prevalence, Behavioral Risks and Mass Media* (Cape Town: HSRC Publishers, 2002); World Health Organization (WHO), *HIV/AIDS Epidemiological Surveillance Report for the WHO African Region. 2005 Update* (Geneva: WHO, 2005)

[3]Anthony Brink, *Debating AZT: Mbeki and the AIDS Drug Controversy* (Pietermaritzburg: Open Books, 2000); Neville Hoad, "Thabo Mbeki's AIDS Blues: The Intellectual, the Archive, and the Pandemic," *Public Culture* 17 (2005): 101-28; Ann Strode, *Understanding the Institutional Dynamics of South Africa's Response to the HIV/AIDS Pandemic* (Pretoria: Idasa, 2000).

[4]Desmond Cohen, *Poverty and HIV/AIDS in Sub-Saharan Africa* (New York: United Nations Development Program, UNDP, 2000); Desmond Cohen, "Joint Epidemics: Poverty and AIDS in Sub-Saharan Africa," *Harvard International Review* 23 (2001): 54-58; Nana K. Poku, "Africa's AIDS Crisis in Context: 'How the Poor are Dying,'" *Third World Quarterly* 22 (2000): 191-204; Alan Whiteside, "Poverty and HIV/AIDS in Africa," *Third World Quarterly* 23 (2002): 313-32.

[5]K. Zuma et al, "Risk Factors of Sexually Transmitted Infections Among Migrant and Non-Migrant Sexual Partnerships from Rural South Africa," *Epidemiology & Infection*, 133 (2005): 421-428.

[6]B. L. Meel, "Incidence of HIV Infection at the Time of Incident Report in Victims of Sexual Assault, Between 2000 and 2004, in Transkei, Eastern Cape, South Africa," *African Health Sciences* 5 (2005): 207-12; Shereen Mills, "Violence Against Women and Children: A Review of South African Studies," *Gender Research Programme Bulletin* 1 (2004); K. Wood, and R. Jewkes, "Violence, Rape, and Sexual Coercion: Everyday Love in a South African Township," *Gender and Development*, 5 (1996): 41-46.

[7]Suzanne Leclerc-Madlala, "Youth, HIV/AIDS and the Importance of Sexual Culture and Context" (Working Paper No. 9, Centre for Social Science Research, University of Cape Town, 2000); Donald Skinner, "How do Youth in Two Communities Make Decisions about Using Condoms?" (Working Paper No. 2, Centre for Social Science Research, University of Cape Town, 2000).

[8]Marlise Richter, "Customary Law, Gender and HIV/AIDS," *Gender Research Programme Bulletin* 1 (2004): 4

[9]Likhapha Ntsoareng-Mbatha, "How Many Wives is Enough?" *Gender Research Programme Bulletin* 1 (1996)

[10]Teresa Mugadza, "Discrimination against Women in the World of Human Rights: The Case of Women in Southern Africa," in *The Handbook of Women, Psychology, and*

the Law, ed. Andreas Barnes (San Francisco: Jossey-Bass, 2005), 354.

[11] R. Jewkes et al., "He must Give Me Money, He Mustn't Beat Me": Violence against Women in three South African Provinces (Pretoria: Medical Research Council, 1999); Charles Wendo, "African Women Denounce Bride Price," The Lancet 363 (2004): 716.

[12] Nicola Ansell, " 'Because it's Our Culture!' (Re)negotiating the Meaning of Lobola in Southern African Secondary Schools," Journal of Southern African Studies 27 (2001): 697-716; Alice K. Armstrong, Culture and Choice: Lessons from Survivors of Gender Violence in Zimbabwe (Harare: Legal Resources Foundation, 2000).

[13] Tabitha T. Langen, "Gender Power Imbalance on Women's Capacity to Negotiate Self-Protection against HIV/AIDS in Botswana and South Africa" African Health Sciences 5 (2005): 188-97.

[14] Anthony C. LoBaido, "Child-Rape Epidemic in South Africa," http://www.worldnetdaily.com/news/article.asp?ARTICLE_ID=25806 (December 26, 2001).

[15] Wendo, "African Women Denounce Bride Price."

[16] Heike Becker, "Researching Gender and Customary Law in Namibia" (paper presented at the Researching Gender and Law Conference, Johannesburg, South Africa, March 15-17, 1996).

[17] Leclerc-Madlala, "Youth, HIV/AIDS and the Importance of Sexual Culture and Context."

[18] Sangoma is a Zulu word meaning "traditional African doctor".

[19] Maretha J. Visser, Johan B. Schoeman, and Jan J. Perold, "Evaluation of HIV/AIDS Prevention in South African Schools," Journal of Health Psychology, 9 (2004): 263-280.

[20] The correlation between the rumors that HIV came from Port Elizabeth and the widespread assertion that homosexuality was openly practiced there does not reflect people's knowledge about HIV epidemiology. Homosexuality was associated with HIV only morally.

[21] Philip Mayer, Townsmen or Tribesmen: Urbanization in a Divided Society (Cape Town: Oxford University Press, 1961).

CHAPTER 4

Navigating the AIDS Epidemic in Rural Malawi[1]

SUSAN COTTS WATKINS

Times are unsettled in rural Malawi. Deaths from a new disease, AIDS, have provoked great uncertainty, as have the accompanying global and national prescriptions of behavior change. Many people are worried about becoming infected. But the prescribed straight-and-narrow channels to safe harbor – abstinence, fidelity, and condoms – are widely considered incompatible with long-standing conceptions of the good life, particularly the joys of sex. Thus, men and women in Malawi are collectively navigating the AIDS epidemic. In conversations with relatives, friends, neighbors, acquaintances, and strangers, they publicly evaluate sources of risk and varieties of sexual pleasure, debate global and national prescriptions, and formulate local, and sometimes innovative, strategies of prevention.

In her book *Talk of Love*, Ann focuses on "culture in action." When times are unsettled, she writes, "people use culture to organize new strategies of action and to model new ways of thinking and feeling ... Individuals in certain phases of their lives, and groups or entire societies at certain historical moments, are involved in constructing new strategies of action."[2] A similar conception of collective change is evident in Paul DiMaggio's "Culture and Cognition," in which he calls for research on the types of social interaction that lead "large numbers of persons rapidly to adopt orientations that might have appeared culturally alien to the majority of them a short time before."[3] Swidler's data come from the United States in recent times, a context that is far less unsettled than contemporary Malawi; DiMaggio's article is theoretical. Both publications, however, provide a useful framework for analyzing responses to AIDS in rural Malawi.

My evidence comes from a rich variety of survey and qualitative data collected in rural Malawi between 1997 and 2004, a period I expect to be, in retrospect, the turning point of the epidemic in Malawi. This prediction contradicts much of the literature on the AIDS epidemic in sub-Saharan Africa, which postulates that "silence and denial" are barriers to the goals of prevention programs that aim to change sexual behavior throughout the continent. This article shows that there is little silence or denial. Whether my prediction of the coming diminution in the epidemic is accurate can only be established in the future through measurements of a decline in the incidence of HIV. The evidence presented below, however, suggests communal cultural change in that direction as well as limits to the power of those outside local social networks to hasten the pace of change.

Below I describe and justify the unusual data on local conversations that I use, and also acknowledge their limitations. I then distinguish three building blocks from which local strategies of behavior are constructed: crucial epidemiological information disseminated by international and national actors; visible evidence of the epidemic provided by deaths from AIDS, which appear to have catalyzed the formulation of local strategies of prevention; and the social construction of sex in rural Malawi. I describe the prevention strategies themselves, which range from the internationally and nationally prescribed abstinence, fidelity, and condom use to innovative strategies of partner selection, divorce, and renewed religious commitment. Although my aim here is to add to our understanding of collective responses to the epidemic in one rural population, I end by considering the extent to which locally formulated strategies of prevention may be effective in altering the course of the epidemic and I speculate about the applicability of my findings to other populations.

Data

My data come from an ongoing project in rural Malawi, the Malawi Diffusion and Ideational Change Project. The quantitative data consist of two rounds of a longitudinal household survey, with an initial sample of approximately 1,500 ever-married women and 1,000 of their husbands (Malawi 1 in 1998, Malawi 2 in 2001).[4] Because these data are of secondary importance here and have been described elsewhere,[5] I do not discuss them. The qualitative data consist of semistructured interviews and field journals kept by local participant-observers. I rely heavily on the latter.

The observational field journals address three problems that our project team encountered and that are probably characteristic of data collection through conventional survey methods or semistructured interviews in similar contexts. The first is that respondents perceive that data collection is funded by the government with support from foreign donors, and they expect material benefit from their participation. Evaluations of our data and of Demographic and Health Survey data led us to suspect that survey respondents thus often shaped their responses toward conformity with the behavioral prescriptions of government programs.[6] This is likely to be the case in other poor countries of sub-Saharan Africa as well.[7] Second, analyses of our survey data showed the importance of characteristics of respondents' social networks for individual responses to AIDS.[8] However, attempts to learn about the content of network conversations through tape-recorded semistructured interviews proved to be unsatisfactory, since retrospective reporting of who said what to whom was usually laconic and subject to the same biases in reporting as the survey data. Third, neither the surveys nor the semistructured interviews permit us to appreciate the dynamism of the conversations as they occurred, with participants adding information or opinions, interrupting each other, agreeing or disagreeing; nor do they show how participants move from particular anecdotes about specific individuals to generalizations about the dangers of the epidemic and to consideration of strategies of prevention.

Thus, we adapted the practices of ethnographers. Rather than import a single educated ethnographer to hang out, observe, and keep field notes, we asked several village residents to do this – to simply recall what they could of conversations about AIDS that they overheard or participated in during their daily lives, and to write their recollections in a journal as soon as possible after the conversation occurred and in as much detail as they could remember. (Later, religion was added as a second topic.) There are approximately 300 journals, covering a period of five years, from August 1999 to September 2004; most of them were written by four local ethnographers. During periods of our fieldwork, the journalists sometimes dictated their recollections of a recent conversation to me. Otherwise, they wrote in common school notebooks, which were mailed through an intermediary in Blantyre. The journalists were not supervised and no journals were rejected, although in a few cases I wrote asking for clarification. The conversations were in local languages in which the journalists are fluent, but they were written in English – and often hastily, such that the grammar is sometimes poor and words omitted. I have corrected the mistakes in grammar and spelling that interfered with legibility.[9]

Although there are few journalists, the number of individuals whose words are recorded in the journals is large. Each journalist interacts frequently with a small number of friends, relatives, and neighbors who know one another; thus, they are members of what network analysts describe as dense networks. These networks are usually homophilous, that is, their members are similar to one another in terms of sex, age, wealth, and education, as is characteristic of social networks in the United States and elsewhere.[10] However, the journalists also interact with or overhear strangers or people known to them only by name, a more heterogeneous category. For example, in a period of five weeks one journalist reported overhearing or talking with 28 people about funerals. She knew some of them well, others by name only, and yet others not at all. She herself attended four funerals, the average attended by female respondents in the 2001 survey round in the previous month. She talked with five relatives of the deceased and four friends and neighbors of the deceased and talked with or overheard five other people she knows by name and 14 she does not know by name. In addition, in previous journals she had talked with three of the deceased, all friends of hers, as they became ill and recognized that they were dying.

The journals display great diversity in natural conversational settings, as illustrated by my summary of one journal (the journalists are identified by a pseudonym and the year):

> The journal begins on the 14th of June, 2001, when the journalist, Alice, visits her cousin, who is a nurse at a hospital about an hour's bus-ride away. The cousin, who is pregnant, tells Alice that three months after her marriage her husband began coughing, then a headache, then diarrhea, then both diarrhea and shingles, all of which involved stays in the hospital. The cousin herself had become thin. The cousin requested that they both be tested, and both were HIV positive. Later, Alice returns for the husband's funeral, where she talks with her cousin and her cousin's mother. The cousin warns Alice, a widow, to be careful whom she marries, and to be sure to have a blood test beforehand. On the way home from the funeral, Alice meets a man at the bus stop who has been to see a brother ill with tuberculosis; he tells her that the TB ward is full, they all have AIDS (presumably including his brother). Another man at the bus stop joins the conversation, asking why it is that women appear to

have AIDS more than men. This generates a lengthy discussion about differences in men's and women's behavior and bodies, whether or not it is possible to use a condom in marriage, medications, and about the history of AIDS, with all of these topics introduced not by the journalist but by the men, none of whom Alice knows. Two weeks later Alice returns for the funeral of her cousin's newborn baby. Walking back from the funeral to the bus stop, a neighbor of her cousin asks Alice why her cousin is so thin, and then comments that people are saying she has AIDS because although she herself was innocent, her husband was promiscuous and, as a woman, she could not refuse to have sex with her husband. On the bus, a woman starts a conversation with Alice about AIDS, which is then joined by the third person on their seat, an old man. Again, the others introduce the topics, which cover AIDS as God's punishment, AIDS as witchcraft, AIDS as a government plot, and AIDS as a result of youth who disobey the advice of their parents. A few weeks later Alice goes to the funeral of her cousin, where she overhears others explaining that her cousin was the innocent victim of her husband. (Alice 2001)

This journal is unusual in consisting primarily of a series of incidents linked by Alice's travels; in contrast, many of the journals consist of five to ten unrelated conversational incidents. It is also unusual in including a participant who is open about her own HIV status; more typically, people identify others as HIV positive, often expressing sympathy as well as empathy. But this journal is also typical of other journals in several ways: the participants in the conversations are not only relatives and friends but also strangers and acquaintances; the discussions often occur in public spaces such as on a bus, in the market, or at a bar (for men) or at the maize mill (for women); and, typically, there are more than two conversational partners. Alice's journal is also typical in that a diversity of views about AIDS are expressed.

Many conversational interactions share a similar structure. The conversation is stimulated by news that a particular person, known at least by name to the others, is ill or has died. The participants jointly construct a "social autopsy," a narrative of the person's sexual and medical history, then evaluate his or her behavior, and finally move from the specific anecdote to generalizations about the epidemic and appropriate strategies for prevention. Considerations of space limit the extent to which I can illustrate the flow of the conversations, but the following provides a truncated example. (In this and subsequent journal illustrations, I use double quotes around the journalist's words and italics when the journalist cites the words of one or more participants; the journalists often used parentheses to indicate an explanatory aside, and I use brackets around my own insertions.)

> Background: The journalist has gone to the trading center [a small market] to buy soap for his wife and fish for lunch. He chats with a fish vendor who is a friend of his and then they both chat with a customer, who has sores on her face. Once she leaves, they are joined by a neighboring vendor who had been listening. Together they diagnose the woman's condition as shingles, which they interpret as a symptom of AIDS. They justify this diagnosis by providing a narrative of her sexual history: she's had four marriages, all ending in divorce because she was unfaithful. They then speculate as to whether her unfaithfulness was due to a need for money for her children, or to lust, and why in these days of the epidemic any man would select her as a sexual partner. One man "went on saying that she is on the way to the graveyard, this is not the time of playing with men by doing sex with them, neither should men be playing with women by doing sex with them. He said that people tend to think that probably there is AIDS in this world but that it only attacks some people. They think they themselves are special, but this is a childish idea. My friend said that of course it might happen that we all have AIDS but we should not be trying to get more and more AIDS viruses, because when you contract AIDS you will be regretting ... Friend continued saying that if one wants to enjoy sex with many partners he should try to use condoms always. Although the government has introduced them and they are distributed free of charge, we neglect to use them. We chatted and chatted and finally we concluded saying that nowadays it's better to just stop going with other sexual partners, it's better that whenever he wants sex he should select a bargirl, because one cannot think of having plain sex with the bargirl. Everyone knows that any bargirl has AIDS and therefore everyone having sex with her protects himself by using condoms ... Finally we all agreed that only an immediate change of behavior will protect us from catching AIDS. We chatted and chatted until I just bought the fish ... " (Simon 2003)

How valid are these data? There are two issues: acting for an audience and the accuracy of the journalists' recollections. It is to be expected that in informal social interactions participants manage their presentation of self, just as they do in the formal contexts of surveys and qualitative interviews. Although these informal presentations of self may not be more "true" than those that occur with an interviewer with clipboard or tape recorder, they are likely to be different – for example, men are presumably more inclined to brag about their sexual conquests to their peers than to an interviewer with a clipboard.[11] Nonetheless, I think statements such as "an immediate change of behavior will protect us" are more credible when made to peers than to an interviewer. In addition, when a participant says something implausible, another participant often challenges it, something interviewers are trained to avoid doing. But for the purposes here, the authenticity of views expressed in conversations is less important than that they are publicly expressed to others, and thus illustrate the diversity of views to which people are exposed in their daily lives.

Just as interviewer error cannot be ignored when assessing survey data, one cannot assume that every journal entry perfectly repeats what was actually said. Some things may have been forgotten, and the journalists may have shaped their writing for what they perceived to be my interests. A potentially more serious issue is falsification. The journalists were paid US$30 for each journal, a substantial amount in a country where per capita income is estimated to be approximately US$170 per year.[12] Thus, it is likely that the journalists spent more time at places, such as the trading center, where they would be likely to overhear conversations about AIDS, than they otherwise would do. But in most of the journal entries the verisimilitude of the narrative and the vivid detail suggest that falsification is unlikely. In addition, cross-checking for consistency across journals provides some reassurance. Some individuals or events appear in the recollections of a single journalist over a period of several years, and some individuals appear in the recollections of more than one journalist. In addition, on some topics there is consistency between the journals, the survey data, and the semistructured interviews. Thus, it is unlikely that the journals are elaborate fictional narratives.

Admittedly, qualitative data are more difficult to summarize succinctly than quantitative data and permit great latitude in the selection of quotes. Because there is much in the literature on AIDS that provides reason for pessimism, here I have taken advantage of this latitude to select journal entries that illustrate what I expect to be successful strategies for confronting AIDS.

Context

Next I briefly describe the building blocks with which rural men and women are constructing strategies of prevention: the information provided by the prevention programs of international and national actors, the timing of the perception in rural communities that AIDS poses a personal risk, and the social construction of sex in rural communities.

International and national prevention activities

Beginning in 1985 global actors projected the spread of an AIDS epidemic in Africa and disseminated information about the epidemiology of HIV. Although rural Malawi has been familiar with sexually transmitted infections (STIs) – for example, gonorrhea and syphilis – at least since colonial times, symptoms of such STIs, if they appear, do so quickly.[13] Thus, the information that the new disease was sexually transmitted and that it was fatal was crucial: the long delay between HIV infection and symptoms would have made it difficult to perceive the connection between sex and death. Global actors also promoted strategies for behavior change – the "ABCs" of prevention (Abstinence, Being faithful after marriage, and Condom use). The information that abstinence, fidelity, and condom use could prevent a sexually transmitted disease was unnecessary. Malawians had long known that these behaviors would prevent STIs, but in the past they were willing to risk infection because they believed that the familiar STIs could be cured. This willingness to risk infection became more costly once it was clear that AIDS has no cure.[14]

Even after a series of information dissemination meetings in Africa in the 1980s, President Kamuzu Banda's government (1963-93) made only modest efforts to respond to the epidemic. After the first official case was diagnosed, blood screening was begun, but there were no notable prevention programs, even in urban areas. Nonetheless, a 1993 survey in the same rural area of southern Malawi in which our project is located showed that 99 percent of both men and women knew that the new disease was sexually transmitted and 96 percent responded that it could not be cured.[15] In addition, the vast majority agreed that one could get AIDS from sex with healthy-looking people and that it was possible to protect oneself from infection.[16] Bakili Muluzi, elected president in 1994, was more publicly open about AIDS. Shortly after his election he led an AIDS march and permitted donors to market condoms and government officials to develop short- and medium-term plans for donors. But only in 2002 did the government finalize an "integrated behavior change intervention strategy,"[17] well after, as I show below, rural Malawians had developed their own strategies.

Estimates of HIV prevalence in Malawi have been stable or declining since 1999. The most recent estimate, for 2003, is that 14 percent of adults aged 15-49 and living outside the major urban areas are infected (UNAIDS 2004).[18] Yet the only intervention programs that appear prominently in local conversations about AIDS are the widespread availability of condoms, prevention messages on the radio, and school-based "Just Say No to AIDS" clubs. Other prevention programs are still few and far between in the rural sites of our project. Even had interventions begun earlier and been more vigorous, however, it is likely that they would have been ineffective until rural Malawians began to hear anecdotes about local people who died of AIDS.

Perceptions of risk

As other writers have pointed out, the long period between infection with HIV and death from AIDS is "key to understanding the difficulties individuals and societies have in recognizing the scale of HIV's threat."[19] The first cases of AIDS were officially diagnosed in 1985, although it is likely that there were some infections earlier.[20] An analysis of Malawi census data shows a marked increase in mortality between 1977 and 1987, but predominantly among children under age ten.[21] An increase in child mortality at that time may not have been attributed to AIDS or even noticed, however, because baseline child mortality was high, and in high-mortality settings child deaths are both expected and variable. Stories about AIDS sufferers appear to have begun circulating in rural Malawi later, in the mid-1990s, when adult neighbors and relatives began to die.[22]

Few people in Malawi or elsewhere in sub-Saharan Africa are tested for HIV, but villagers collectively and confidently diagnose AIDS on the basis of social autopsies that combine local knowledge of the progression of the sufferer's symptoms with local knowledge of his or her sexual history. Some argue about the cause of death, especially when the deceased is a relative, and attribute it to illnesses with similar symptoms.[23] However, when our survey respondents were asked, "If someone was thin and died, what would you think he/she died from?," more than 90 percent said AIDS. In the field journals the symptoms are more detailed (e.g., loss of weight, diarrhea, skin diseases, and, especially, failure to respond to treatment). The sexual history is also often quite specific, including a chronological narrative of the sexual partners of the deceased, as well as the decedent's partners' partners and whether they were now dead, ill, or well. Because symptoms and sexual biographies are the stuff of gossip in the community and thus well known, the socially constructed diagnoses are probably fairly accurate. Even if they are not, what is relevant here is the public perception that so-and-so died of AIDS and the implications of that diagnosis for those who hear the stories.

Those who witnessed relatives, friends, and neighbors dying of AIDS were clearly unsettled and talked with emotion about their experience. For some, the experience appears to have been a catalyst for behavior change. In one incident, a young man tells several friends that he has reformed his behavior. They ask why, and he explains:

> "Only because I have seen for myself, some of my friends have died because of this disease AIDS, and I do care for my life. AIDS troubles a lot! I didn't say anything. He kept on, saying, For example, there was a certain army pensioner who was living up there in my village ... He was very sick indeed, going to the hospital, no treatment, private hospitals – just wasting money and then he came home and was sick until he became like a very little young child. I was going to see him during the whole course of his suffering. You could liken him to a two-year-old child when he lay down sick ... And the way I had seen him suffering, that's when I came to my senses, that indeed AIDS troubles a great deal before one dies." (Simon 2002)

The young man attributes his behavior change to seeing a neighbor who he knew had many sex partners decline physically, but we know from other journals that this witness had himself been promiscuous. Thus, it is likely that while watching his neighbor waste away he imagined himself as "a two-year-old child." We do not know whether the reforms he claimed to have made happened at all, or persisted, or occurred too late. We do know that many in Malawi have had similar experiences watching those with whom they can identify die, as well as hearing about other deaths they did not witness. If we are persuaded by the literature in psychology that "people disproportionately weight *salient, memorable* or *vivid* evidence even when they have better sources of information,"[24] then anecdotes about people who are known in the community are likely to provide particularly compelling motivations for change.

The joys of sex

Given such motivation, why doesn't behavior change occur more speedily? Below I describe the cultural process occurring in rural Malawi as social networks reconsider the preventive measures they have long known can prevent sexually transmitted infections in the face of a new, and fatal, sexually transmitted infection. The dissemination of epidemiological information about the new disease and the increasing numbers of deaths occurred in a context in which both women and men say that frequent sex is important and that the joys of sex are diminished by condoms; in addition, men talk enthusiastically about the pleasures of multiple partners, boasting that "my girlfriends could fill a Yanu-Yanu bus."[25] Whether or not sex is actually frequent or nonmarital sexual partners are common cannot be known. As I noted earlier, self-reports on such behavior on surveys are likely to be flawed, and perhaps the same is true in conversational interactions. However, frank talk about the importance of sexual satisfaction seems to be common rather than taboo, both in our data and in research by others.[26]

The language of taste is used by both men and women in talking about sex: it is so "sweet" that a common objection to condom use is that "you can't taste the sweetness," "it's like eating sweets in a wrapper." Deviations from an expected frequency of sex, for example because of postpartum abstinence or geographical separation, have long justified adultery in Malawi, and this remains true today.[27] A case at a chief's court illustrates this point. A woman sought a divorce because she had discovered her husband *in flagrante* with her neighbor. The husband, wife, and counselors for each party made their case to the chief and to the audience that had assembled under a large tree. As the plaintiff related her story, she said:

> "It's not this time that one should be tolerating this bad tendency, there is AIDS and if he has already given me the disease then I will not mind, I am still going home, I will die in my parent's house." The audience murmured sympathetically. However, when the husband testified that his wife had refused sex for a week, so he needed "to be relieving my agonies and sexual desires the woman [his wife]

was refusing," the journalist commented that "some faint murmurings were to be heard in the audience that the man did well and he could not do otherwise if the spouse was refusing to sleep with him." The chief's summation features President Muluzi's concerns about AIDS, but in the end he decrees that the couple should reconcile. (Simon 2002)

Men say that multiple partners are desirable because each woman is different: just as "You can't eat only *nsima* every day" (*nsima*, made from cornmeal, is the staple food), you can't be satisfied with just one woman. In addition, having multiple partners signals masculinity.[28] Sexual desire also leads wives to engage in extramarital encounters. In interviews conducted with a subsample of our survey respondents, Linda Tawfik found that a common motivation for married women's adultery is that their husbands do not satisfy them sexually.[29]

Older rural Malawians are nostalgic about the good old days when sex could be enjoyed and diseases risked because they could be cured. The incident described below occurred among three relatives in a bar, one of whom points to three men with a prostitute:

> "And he said, Y*ou see those men, they are drinking with a prostitute and at the end one of them will go for her. That's no enjoyment in these days as there is AIDS. The good days were those when we were young men. We are the ones who enjoyed women freely because in those days we were just afraid of some sexually transmitted diseases that were curable like buboes, gonorrhea, and syphilis and all these were getting treated. Just imagine how people are dying of AIDS these days."* (Diston 2002)

Now, even men too young to have experienced the golden age mourn the lost joys of sex and are struggling to find acceptable compromises.

Strategies of prevention

Table 4.1 uses data from the first two rounds of the longitudinal survey conducted by the Malawi Diffusion and Ideational Change Project. Although the sample was designed to represent the rural areas of three specific districts, comparison with the rural population of the Malawi Demographic and Health Surveys shows that our sample is reasonably representative of the national rural population.[30] The 1998 sample consists of ever-married women aged 15-49 and their husbands of all ages; in this table, however, husbands and wives are not linked.

Table 4.1 shows that rural Malawians are – not surprisingly, given the number of funerals they attend – worried about AIDS. Men are less worried than women, a consistent finding in surveys in sub-Saharan Africa.[31] Husbands may have a greater sense of invulnerability than wives because they are more likely to believe that they have taken steps to prevent AIDS by changing their extramarital behavior, whereas wives may perceive they have less control over whether or not they become infected by their husband. Table 4.1 also shows that the proportion worried about infection has declined, a reduction that is associated with several of the strategies of prevention described below.[32] Particularly interesting is that respondents vastly overestimate the transmission probabilities of HIV. Although most of the respondents report that sex only once with an infected person is certain to lead to infection, epidemiologists estimate the probabilities as much lower, approximately three sexual acts in a thousand in contexts such as rural Malawi where untreated STIs, some of which are known to be co-factors for HIV transmission, are common.[33] The field journals show that in addition to overestimating transmission probabilities, people vastly underestimate the duration from infection to symptoms of AIDS.

Although almost everyone knows AIDS is sexually transmitted and, thus, like the STIs long known in rural Malawi, can be prevented by strict abstinence, fidelity, and condom use, in the past it was possible to risk infections that could be cured. In the face of the new sexually transmitted infection, it is understood that such complacency is no longer warranted. There remains, however, great uncertainty about how to prevent infection in ways that still permit the joys of sex. The navigational charts for avoiding AIDS that are officially promoted are unattractive: thus the search for modified or alternative channels.

Below I begin with fidelity, which is considered to be a desirable safe harbor in the abstract, but understood to be extremely difficult to reach in practice. Next I discuss the local compromises – a reduction in the number of partners and a more careful selection of partners – strategies that are considered to permit sexual pleasure outside of marriage while reducing the likelihood of infection. I then turn to condom use, which is currently perceived as a particularly unattractive strategy and certainly not

Table 4.1: **Risk perceptions, 1998 and 2001, women and men, rural Malawi**[a]

	Women		Men	
	1998	2001	1998	2001
	N= 878	N= 878	N= 675	N= 675
Worried about getting AIDS (%)				
Very worried	61	49	52	37
Moderately worried	22	26	21	21
Not at all worried	17	26	27	42
Perceived risk				
Risk of acquiring AIDS[b](%)				
None	n/a	32	n/a	48
Some		64		50
Don't know		5		2
Likelihood of being infected already (%)				
None	n/a	54	n/a	69
Low		19		16
Medium		7		5
High		9		3
Don't know		11		6
Likelihood of infection if one has				
sex once with infected person (%)				
None/low	n/a	3	n/a	3
High		30		29
Certain		67		68
Social interactions				
Know someone who died of AIDS[c] (%)	96	98	96	98
Number of persons known				
who died of AIDS (median)[d]	5	5	5	6
Number of funerals attended in last month				
0	n/a	4	n/a	5
1-3		49		37
4-6		31		38
7+		16		21
Median		3		4
At least one network partner worried	90	84	87	81

n/a = not available because question was not asked.

NOTE: The sample used for this table is smaller than the total sample because it includes only respondents for whom data are available from both survey rounds, except for those questions that were only asked in the second survey round.

[a] The women in the sample were between ages 15-49 in 1998. The men are husbands of these women, with no restriction by age.

[b] Respondents reports of the likelihood that they currently have or in the future will have AIDS.

[c] Calculated from a question regarding the number of acquaintances suspected to have died of AIDS.

[d] Excludes respondents who answered "dont know" (32 in 1998, 19 in 2001).

SOURCE: Kirsten P. Smith, and Susan C. Watkins, "Perceptions of Risk and Strategies for Prevention: Responses to HIV/AIDS in Rural Malawi," *Social Science & Medicine* 60 (2005): 649-660.

appropriate within marriage. I discuss fidelity and its adaptations first, because these strategies are far more important in conversations within social networks than are other strategies; an emphasis on fidelity is also far more attractive to the government of Malawi, as it has been to governments elsewhere in sub-Saharan Africa. Lastly, I examine the particular tensions within marriage. Rural spouses have by now come to understand that their fates are joined: even if one spouse is faithful, the other may not be.

Fidelity

The literature on AIDS in sub-Saharan Africa might leave the impression that no man is faithful. This is unlikely. Fidelity is preached by the Christian and Muslim religions to which most of our respondents belong, and is particularly central to the doctrines of the rapidly increasing Evangelical and Pentecostal denominations.[34] There are other reasons as well to expect that some are faithful, such as satisfaction with one's spouse or low libido.

As shown in Table 4.1, a substantial proportion of survey respondents are not worried about the possibility of becoming infected. How could this be? The semistructured interviews we conducted in 1999 suggest that those who are not worried believe, probably rightly, that they have little reason to worry. An analysis of these interviews showed that only 7 out of 64 husbands and 3 out of 64 wives said they had not discussed AIDS with their spouses.[35] Some wives who claimed to have had no discussions were convinced that their husband was faithful, even in the face of aggressive probing by the interviewer as illustrated below (the respondent's words are italicized; the female respondent is identified by her survey ID):

> Respondent: *That one's heart is the same as mine....* Interviewer: How do you know? R: *Ah, I see him.* I: Mmmm. R: *Yes, because if a person is doing this and that, it is easy to see him.* I: Just to see a person, you can know his heart? R: *Yes, of course, because I got married to him long ago but I never heard anything.* I: You never heard anything about him? R: *I never heard and I never saw him going here and there.* (ID 6039)

Those who believe their spouse to be faithful may be deceiving themselves or may be reluctant to voice suspicions to an interviewer. Yet one spouse can rather easily monitor the behavior of the other. For example, a wife knows when her husband comes home late, or not at all, and can interpret his disinterest in intercourse with her as an indication that he is finding satisfaction elsewhere. In addition, our qualitative data (the field journals as well as several sets of interviews conducted for dissertations with subsamples of survey respondents) show that both women and men are very likely to learn about their spouse's infidelity from friends, relatives, or neighbors who report suspicious behavior to them.[36]

Some respondents say fidelity is simply impossible to achieve and thus all will die, elaborating that a) God made humans, b) humans like sex, c) therefore sex is God-given and should not, perhaps cannot, be constrained. Others say that faithfulness is possible for those who are not faithful by nature or socialization, but it is very difficult to achieve. In one journal entry, a young man tells others that after getting a sexually transmitted infection he realized that if he continued with promiscuous behavior he would also get AIDS:

> *"Life is very important and we need not be playing with life, it can't be bought when it is lost."* The journalist wrote that initially the young man tried masturbating when he was away from his regular partner, but gave that up because he lost weight. He stopped drinking beer, since when he was drunk, he looked for partners. He spoke to the journalist about temptation: *"Nowadays young girls are dressing very attractively and need money and if you are not careful you may end up contracting AIDS because you cannot resist the temptations exerted by these girls pertaining to their attractive dressings."* (Simon 2001)

The temptations are somewhat different for wives. They are usually portrayed in the Western media and in donor policy statements as "vulnerable women" who need money for basic necessities. But some also turn to other partners in exchange for luxuries such as lotions, or because their husbands are not satisfying them sexually, or because they are seeking revenge for their husbands' infidelity.[37]

One innovative solution to the difficulties of achieving fidelity is seeking support in religion. Religion is infrequently included in studies of AIDS-related behavior, and, when it is, the categories of religious denominations are crude, typically only Catholic, Protestant, and Muslim. Yet the observational journals provide indications that conversion to a spirit-type denomination or becoming born again within a mainline denomination may have attractions for those seeking support for resisting temptations that might bring them death:[38]

"Then my friend Davis said, *I have come to realize now, friend, that
we are just playing in this world while others are really fighting hard
to reach God, to inherit another life in future after this life and live
again in another good life in heaven.* And I said frankly to him,
Friend! I am very startled to hear what you are saying now. Why
have you decided to think like this yet every time we chat ... you say
you like having sex with ladies and you enjoy the game, so how are
you going to deal with this? He answered, *I am saying this because
my friend Moses has written me a letter, once again telling me that he
is married now and left all the childish wickedness he was doing. He
also said he is now working at a hospital department and is still Born
Again, and he gave me many verses to read about the importance of
marrying ... After I scientifically considered what he wrote, and read
for myself the verses in the Bible he gave me, I realized that I have
been wasting my time messing around with girls who might destroy
my life instead of changing my behavior and marrying.* And I mocked
him: Then you are to be a Born Again and marry and be living in a
faithful life because of your friend? Then my friend said, *Not that,
but I believe it is because of time, my time has just come for me to
be a Born Again, marry, have children and head the family.*" (Simon
2002)

There is some reason to believe that religious conviction may reduce
the risk of AIDS. Gregson et al. found in a study in Zimbabwe that HIV
prevalence is lower in the spirit-type denominations in which marital fidelity is a central tenet than in mainline Christian denominations.[39] An
analysis of our 2001 survey data showed that a third of those who reported
being born again had converted in 1996 or subsequently, consistent with
the timing of the recognition that AIDS had reached the villages.[40] Pi-
lot interviews with some of these respondents showed that for some, the
dense and encompassing social networks of spirit-type denominations are
perceived as supporting one's efforts to resist the temptations of multiple
sexual partners, consistent with characterizations in the literature of born-
again networks as providing a "security circle," a "defensive 'wall' against
outside evil forces ..."[41]

Compromises with fidelity

Because sex is perceived as central to the good life, because a variety of
sexual partner is considered to add spice to life, and because resisting temp-

tation is understood to be so difficult, modifications of fidelity are the main strategies of prevention being discussed in local networks. The primary modifications are a reduction in the number of partners, a more careful selection of partners, and the use of condoms with partners considered to be risky. All are advocated and all are criticized. The reduction in the number of partners is usually interpreted as having only one extramarital partner at a time. The perceived advantages of this strategy are that it provides at least some variety, as well as a source of sexual satisfaction when lengthy abstinence is enjoined, such as after the birth of a child. The critics of this view fall into two camps: those who claim that the sacrifice of greater variety is too great and those who claim that in this era of AIDS any sexual partnership is risky.

Partner selection is a second key strategy. Those who choose their partners carefully are perceived to have a good chance of avoiding infection, whereas those who have sex "anyhow" – indiscriminately – are likely to "catch AIDS." In the following incident a man tells his brother-in-law, a friend, and a schoolteacher that he was caught with a partner postcoitally. This leads to a discussion of various girls in that village and the diseases there, of partner selection, and of condom use. When asked whether he is worried about AIDS, the man laughs and says:

> "I don't overdo it, I only have one partner and after that I go to another partner. And I select them, I don't go anyhow as others there do. Robert then asked, *AIDS has a choice?* He said, *Yes, even when you enter into a shop one chooses the kind of clothes, for example, which might suit him, and their durability.* We laughed...." (Simon 2002)

There is vigorous debate, however, over the criteria for partner selection.[42] Some insist that young and single women are safer partners, either because they have been less sexually active or because they have been more exposed to AIDS prevention messages through the school anti-AIDS clubs. Other participants, however, counter that since the young girls of today are promiscuous and have probably been infected by their teachers, it is better to select older married women, who, they believe, are less likely to be infected. Some also argue that unattractive women are safer, as they are less likely to have multiple partners.

Not having sex "anyhow" is also considered important for women. Although women are not expected to refuse sex with a husband or to insist on condoms with a sexual partner, both men and women grant women considerable autonomy in beginning or ending a relationship:

> *"Every girl or woman is supposed to be proposed to and it's up to her to accept or not."* (Simon 2003)

(Adam Ashforth also makes this point for sexual relationships in Soweto, South Africa.)[43]

Fundamental to the strategy of partner selection is the local knowledge used to diagnose AIDS. As shown earlier in Table 4.1, respondents know that one cannot tell whether someone is infected just by looking: other data are required. Because there is so much gossip in the villages, those who are considering a particular partner may already know a great deal about that person, and, if not, they search for information by asking others. Those who do not consult local knowledge are considered foolish. At the funeral of a village headman, one of our journalists overheard a man identified only by his blue shirt explaining that the headman had married a prostitute whose former husband was repatriated from South Africa because of AIDS, and subsequently died.

> *"If he loved her, he would have asked some people who know her properly about her behavior and he could not have married her, but it has shown that he did not ask anybody else about the woman, he just loved her and proposed to her for the marriage. The woman did not refuse because she knew that if she refuses, nobody will marry her since they know her behavior ..."* (Alice 2003)

Condoms

In Malawi, as elsewhere, there is an exuberant litany of objections to condoms: the condoms themselves are infected, they cause sores on the penis, they come off inside the woman, it is a sin to kill innocent children.[44] Our data on women's attitudes toward condom use are less rich than those on men's attitudes, but it appears that both men and women consider condoms to inhibit the enjoyment of sex. Similar objections to condoms are widespread throughout southern Africa.[45]

In the early journals when condoms were advised, it was typically in a rote manner – "one should use condoms" – and often attributed to messages heard on the radio. This is in stark contrast to recent journals in which conversational partners talk about others', or even their own, use of condoms. Moreover, the illness and sexual history narratives now sometimes end with the moral that failing to use a condom with a prostitute is deliberately choosing death. A female journalist overheard three men talking about the promiscuity of a deceased:

> "One of the men said, *Had it been that she was using condoms, she could not have died today,* and that he knows she wasn't using condoms because his friend, a Medical Assistant at the Health Centre, told him the woman had other sexually transmitted infections. The men then talk about womanizers in general, and a particular driver they know who has AIDS. One of the men says that drivers are *foolish people. They know that there are some condoms which protect people from any disease which one gets from having sex with one who has the disease.* But when men travel and see beautiful women, they are *tantalized by them. They must buy the condoms and carry them wherever else they go. They must use them always and not just having sex with a woman you don't know without using a condom. Look where the problem and loss is. That driver slept with a woman somewhere who was already infected with AIDS and he got it from her at the same time he gave her some money or any other gift which means he bought the AIDS disease for himself. Because of buying AIDS, he bought the painfulness of the disease and he also bought death."* (Alice 2001)

For condom use as for partner selection, local knowledge is critical. Condom use is acceptable with risky partners but not with all partners; thus, one must rely on local knowledge to identify those whose sexual histories render them risky.

It would be desirable to track changes in condom use through survey data, but, as I noted earlier, the validity of survey reports on behavior prescribed by government programs is questionable. Nonetheless, it is striking that on a variety of measures in our survey – condom use for family planning, for extramarital affairs, by "best friend," and by network partners – condom use has increased in every one.[46] In addition to condoms distributed free through clinics, a very rapid increase in condom sales has taken place in Malawi, as elsewhere in the "AIDS belt."[47] This is not to say that objections to condom use have disappeared from local discussions of prevention strategies. Condoms are still a contentious issue and certainly not acceptable within marriage; they remain a foreign "intruder" in the domestic sphere.[48] Condom use within marriage, however, may become more acceptable, much as attitudes toward condom use outside marriage appear to have changed.

Marital strategies

Partner selection is perceived to be particularly important at the time of marriage. It is deeply worrying to many respondents that careful selection of a spouse is not sufficient protection. The advice from prevention programs is directed at individuals. But after marriage it is not sufficient to behave in a way that protects oneself; each spouse is potentially at risk of infection by the other. Moreover, because survey respondents vastly overestimate the probabilities of HIV transmission, they take it for granted that if one spouse is infected the other will also be; both will then die and their children will suffer.

Table 4.2 shows that, especially among women, a substantial proportion consider their primary threat of AIDS to come from a spouse (the high proportion of women reporting "other partner" in 1998 is probably due to a misunderstanding of the question, such that wives meant their husband's "other partner"). Men are also concerned about their wife's fidelity, although they are far less likely to report their suspicion on the surveys or to discuss it in informal conversations with friends, perhaps because men (more than women) are expected to divorce an unfaithful wife.[49]

That women are rightly concerned by the risk they face from a spouse is supported by an analysis of our survey data. Although only a small proportion of husbands reported having an extramarital partner in the past 12 months, there was a statistically significant association between these reports and their wives' reports that their husbands were unfaithful.[50] Another analysis of our data showed that even when the husband's other partner was a co-wife, the co-wife's entry into or exit from the marriage between the 1998 and 2001 surveys affected the respondent's degree of worry.[51] If a 1998 respondent gained a co-wife, she was more than three times as likely to become more worried about HIV/AIDS as women who did not gain a co-wife. In contrast, if a co-wife exited the marriage, the 1998 respondent was twice as likely to become less worried than polygamously married women who did not lose a co-wife between waves.

Currently two strategies are under consideration for dealing with the threat from a spouse: one is to persuade the spouse to be faithful, the other

Table 4.2: Marital relationship as a source of concern, 1998 and 2001, women and men, rural Malawi[a]

| | Women | | Men | |
	1998 N= 878	2001 N= 878	1998 N= 675	2001 N= 675
Percent married[b]	92	92	100	98
Percent polygynous[c]	23	23	14	17
Source of possible infection of greatest concern				
Spouse	32	52	14	23
Other partner	49	20	64	38
Nonsexual (injections/ transfusions/other)	19	28	22	39
Opinion of fidelity of spouse				
Knows/suspects unfaithful	28	27	7	4
Can't/don't know spouse's behavior	21	27	15	16
Probably faithful	51	46	78	80

NOTE: See Note to Table 4.1.
[a] The women in the sample were between ages 15-49 in 1998. The men are husbands of these women, with no restriction by age.
[b] Includes separated respondents.
[c] Restricted to respondents married or separated in both survey rounds.
SOURCE: Smith and Watkins, "Perceptions of risk and strategies for prevention".

is divorce. Because conversations reported in the journals rarely mention spousal conversations, I draw here primarily on an analysis by Eliya Zulu and Gloria Chepngeno of semistructured interviews members of our project team conducted in 1999 with a subsample of our 1998 survey respondents.[52] I focus on the data on women, because women in our surveys report greater concern about their spouse's infidelity than do men, and because the data I present below show that wives are less vulnerable than they are often depicted: rather, they actively use conversations with their spouse and recourse to divorce to protect themselves from infection.

Only nine of the 128 husbands and wives said they had not had a conversation with their spouse about AIDS. The conversations often began much as do the other conversations about AIDS, with news or an anecdote. Then a personally salient moral was drawn: husband and wife must be faithful to each other for the sake of their children. The conversations ended with each assuring the other of his or her commitment to fidelity. Even in the laconic reports to an interviewer who is taping her words, the wife's plea can be quite moving:

Myself, I said ... that you are seeing your friends are dying leaving the children. Is it good that your children should also be suffering like this? Because if it has affected one [spouse], killed one, the other is also finishing [dying] ... So there is nobody to care for the children here on earth. Ah! We are seeing our friends dying – how they are dying. In our family, our sisters, our brothers – they have all finished, leaving children – orphans. (ID 106009)

The recorded conversations between spouses are characterized by considerable diplomacy: only rarely does a wife accuse her husband of infidelity – even when the woman has told the interviewer in an aside that she did not believe her husband's commitment to fidelity.

A more drastic – and innovative – approach than persuasion is divorce. Divorce rates are higher in Malawi than in other sub-Saharan countries for which these rates can be calculated.[53] Just as women have the right to refuse sexual proposals or to end an informal sexual relationship, women have long had rights to initiate divorce under specified circumstances.[54] Currently one of these circumstances is that the woman fears that her husband, by his behavior, will "bring AIDS into the family." It is not clear yet whether fear of infection has increased divorce rates, although our survey data show that the perception that divorce is justified as a protection against infection has increased. In 1998, 16 percent of women agreed that divorce was justified if a woman believed her husband had AIDS; in 2001, 28 percent agreed. But divorce is more difficult than persuasion. It involves assets, including access to land and children, and most think it necessary to justify divorce to their relatives and, in some cases, in a court proceeding.

I illustrate the point with a long excerpt of a conversation among older women. It has the same standard features and themes of the interviews analyzed by Zulu and Chepngeno, as well as the conversations recorded in the journals.

One day while the journalist was babysitting his children, his mother [who lives in the same compound] was visited by a friend who told her that Abiti [Mrs.] Jones had died. His mother shouts the news to the journalist, who comes over, along with two neighbors who also heard her shout. They call the cause of death AIDS, noting that Abiti Jones had twice been hospitalized with TB and that she was faithful but her husband was not. The conversation then turns to generalizations about men and women that make divorce a necessary strategy for women:

"Her friend (my mother's friend) said that, Indeed the late [deceased] was faithful, but the husbands we keep on marrying are killing us because they are the ones who migrate, cheating us that they are going away for business, but they will be sleeping with women there and bringing AIDS to us and we will be dying because of love ... At first they agree that most women just accept whatever her husband brings to them ... Women were born with a silly heart, because most of the time you really know that your husband is running a love affair with such and such a woman but you just keep on being jealous and frowning over him or fighting with the other woman which doesn't help at all. Then a neighbor said that indeed nowadays it's very dangerous and she said that she even tells her husband that whenever she will discover that he has another partner besides her she will certainly divorce him because there is AIDS around ... She tells her husband that if he is tired of her or he had seen that he had overused her and he is fed up with her, it's better to mention that and separate from each other very smartly rather than being double-crossed. [If he] brings AIDS in her family she will be suffering, they will leave the children in great troubles, no one can care for them as well as their parents. The other neighbor said that whenever you come to know that your husband is being promiscuous it's better to talk to him and persuade him to change immediately, but if he does not then divorce will be a good resolution and unquestionable anywhere, even in court, for everyone now is aware that there is AIDS ..." (Simon 2003)

It is very likely that at least some elements of this discussion were repeated to, and then discussed by, other residents, as the news of the death spread and villagers went to the funeral.

An appropriate end to my assessment of women's strategies is a court case in which a woman petitioned for divorce. The chief ruled in favor of the woman and then told the woman and those who were listening:

"Woman, be free and do what seems good to you and to what you believe, you are a brilliant and courageous woman. I congratulate you, keep it up, such kind of behavior, that by doing that you are trying to teach stupid men a lesson as well as protecting yourself from this deadly disease AIDS and also protecting the lives of others like children and those who will marry you in the future." (Simon 2002)

Other strategies

Other innovative but idiosyncratic strategies occasionally appear in the qualitative data. For men, these include reducing sexual desire by soaking a towel in hot water and sleeping with it on the groin, or, in the daytime, exercise or masturbation, or drinking so much that one is unable to have sex. Another prescription is to keep busy, but this is challenged by others who point out that the rich are some of the busiest people, yet they are the ones most likely to have AIDS. It is also noteworthy that some strategies reported in the media are *not* mentioned: for example, in none of our qualitative sources does anyone suggest that having sex with a baby or a virgin would cure AIDS.

Discussion

This article has provided a perspective on "culture in action" in rural Malawi during the unsettled times following the recognition by couples that AIDS was no longer simply an abstract threat to others but a profound danger to themselves and their children. The perspective is social rather than individual, and the primary data are unusual: observational field journals of the conversations of men and women as they discuss whether, and, particularly how, they can successfully navigate the storm of the epidemic. These conversations often feature anecdotes about people much like the participants and often known to them. Together, participants in the conversation collectively and publicly describe the symptoms and the sexual history of an individual, provide explanations for the behavior, and draw a moral from the outcome. Conversations among peers about an illness or death, a couple caught red-handed, or a court case are, I think, far more likely to contribute to normative change than the adventures of soap-opera characters who come to grief because they failed to use a condom.

Our data may be considered problematic when evaluated by sociologists' standards of good survey research and by anthropologists' standards of good ethnography. They do, however, permit us to glimpse diverse and innovative strategies of prevention, including those that are not on the agendas of intervention programs. Participants in conversations with friends, relatives, and neighbors as well as with strangers hear claims that infection is unavoidable and other claims that avoiding infection is possible but very difficult. When some participants point out that persons known to be promiscuous have died, others respond that some who are known to be equally promiscuous have escaped. Similarly, although local knowledge is considered important in selecting sexual partners, there are debates about whether young single partners are less risky than older ones or whether the converse is true. Some of what is said in these local social networks supports pessimistic predictions of the future course of the epidemic, but this article has also pointed to reasons for optimism.

A critical building block for the formulation of local strategies of prevention is the epidemiological information provided by global and national experts, namely that AIDS is sexually transmitted and invariably fatal. That AIDS is transmitted sexually is unlikely to have been uncovered so quickly by rural Malawians on their own, given the long duration between infection and symptoms; and it would have taken time to discover, by trial and error, the lack of efficacy of measures intended as therapeutic. By now, these epidemiological facts are rarely challenged. In contrast, the strict prevention prescriptions – abstinence before marriage, fidelity after, and, if these are unacceptable, consistent condom use – are noisily challenged. In their networks, men and women are collectively modifying the stern prescriptions to make them more compatible with preexisting notions of the good life and are exploring new channels that are not on international or national navigational charts, such as seeking social support in religious communities for resisting temptation, divorcing a partner believed to be infected, or selecting less attractive women as sexual partners.

Rural networks navigating the AIDS epidemic consider fidelity to be a more hospitable safe harbor than consistent condom use. Although it is likely that substantial proportions of couples are indeed faithful, some consider strict fidelity to be a fundamental contradiction to views of the good life, in which the joys of sex are enhanced by a variety of sexual partners. Thus, the strategies of prevention that dominate the discussions of men – the category for whom our data on the content of conversations are more abundant – focus not on strict fidelity, but on compromises: a reduction in the number of extramarital partners and, especially, more deliberate and careful attention to their selection. In selecting partners, it is considered common sense to gather as much local knowledge as possible about the previous behavior of the potential partner, and his or her previous partners as well. Condom use is far less attractive than fidelity or its modifications. The litanies of objections are abundant, ranging from arguments that they are ineffective to arguments that only sex that is "flesh to flesh" is satisfying. Yet there are also signs of change: stories in which the moral point is that so-and-so "deliberately chose death" because he was promiscuous but did not use condoms, or stories about another who escaped infection because he did use condoms. That this new acceptability of condoms is being translated into action is suggested by an increase in condom sales and, perhaps less reliably, by increased survey reports of condom use.

The risk of infection from a spouse is perceived as particularly troublesome. There are few signs of change in the unacceptability of condom use in marriage; but just as attitudes to condom use with extramarital partners appear to have changed, so attitudes toward their use within marriage may change as well.[55] Currently, the preferred strategies for avoiding infection by a spouse are to try to persuade a spouse to be faithful or to divorce a spouse who threatens to bring AIDS into the family. Divorce has long been a solution to marital problems in Malawi; now fear of AIDS is a new rationale. The impression that divorce is an increasingly effective strategy is supported by an increase in the proportion of respondents who say divorce is justified when one partner suspects the other of being infected.

Much humanitarian effort and donor funding have gone into interventions to stem the AIDS epidemic. The interventions have not been demonstrably effective, in part simply because they are rarely rigorously evaluated. Are the local strategies of prevention I have described as under consideration in local networks likely to fare any better? It is not my aim to evaluate their effectiveness, which in any case could only be done with biomarkers measuring the incidence of HIV and other sexually transmitted infections. However, some local strategies are likely to be effective in the aggregate, if not for particular individuals. Rural Malawians are likely to evaluate effectiveness in terms of specific anecdotes: who got infected and why, who escaped and why. Similarly, although public health advocates appear to want to protect every individual, without a vaccine this could be accomplished only if each and every individual complied perfectly with the ABCs of prevention – which is unlikely. Yet, however moving the stories of individuals dying of AIDS, an epidemic is not individual but communal-transmission probabilities matter. For HIV transmission, these probabilities are low. The adoption of fidelity by the uninfected, perhaps as a result of religious conversion or a conversation with a spouse that emphasizes the fate of their children, is certain to be effective in the aggregate, even if not everyone manages to be faithful – or to persuade a spouse to be faithful – all the time. Similarly, the reduction in the number of extramarital partners improves the odds, probably especially when accompanied by more careful partner selection, and is particularly crucial at the time of marriage.[56] People may make mistakes in selecting partners, but avoiding potential partners with risky sexual histories is likely to be better than not consulting social networks to gain such local knowledge. Persuading a spouse to be faithful may work for some, and divorcing an infected spouse is probably effective, even more so if it is not followed by remarriage to another infected person.[57]

The primary data used here are unusual, and Malawi may be unusual as well. How likely is it that similar communal changes are underway elsewhere in sub-Saharan Africa? It is difficult to know, in part because the literature tends to be judgmental and pessimistic: the emphasis is on noncompliance with strict program prescriptions and on "cultural barriers to change," rather than on innovative strategies or "culture in action." Yet there are suggestions that the same processes may be going on elsewhere.

I described three building blocks that served as a foundation for local strategies of prevention: basic epidemiological information about AIDS, the widely discussed appreciation of the joys of sex, and the increase in adult mortality locally attributed to AIDS that I think served as a catalyst for attempts to cope with the epidemic. The first two of these imply similarities in the strategies of prevention likely to be considered elsewhere; the third suggests differences in timing of local prevention efforts. First, the critical epidemiological knowledge appears to be similar in many countries, which is not surprising given the role of global donors in disseminating information.[58] In addition, populations elsewhere in high-prevalence countries had experience with STIs in colonial times[59] and would have known the ABCs of prevention – although, as in Malawi, the availability of effective treatment would have meant that the ABCs did not have to be strictly followed. Lacunae in knowledge – overestimation of HIV transmission probabilities and underestimation of the duration from infection to symptoms – also appear elsewhere.[60] Second, the joys of sex are described similarly in other countries in the region. The connection between sex and food is made elsewhere, and the litanies of objections to condom use elsewhere are similar.[61] The third building block, increases in adult mortality locally attributed to AIDS, is likely to differ across countries in timing, depending largely on when rapid increases in AIDS mortality occurred. Where an increase in adult deaths is great enough to be noticeable, fatalism and denial are unlikely to persist, either in the government or in the population. Other analysts have also argued that "widespread changes in behavior are unlikely to be seen until the impact of HIV-1 infections on morbidity and mortality is clearly visible, and is recognized, and acknowledged by the local population."[62]

Despite similarities in the epidemiological knowledge base, in open appreciation of the joys of sex, or even in the timing of the increase in AIDS-related mortality, one might expect that elsewhere the strategies of prevention in response to the epidemic would differ from the responses in Malawi – for example, in communities where people are more discreet about their sex lives so that local knowledge is skimpy, or divorce had previously been less frequent as a solution to marital problems. Yet there are striking similarities. Men elsewhere also appear to have formulated strategies of fewer partner and more careful selection.[63] Wives' suspicions of their husbands' infidelity are widespread, and an examination of data from the World Health Organization/ Global Program on AIDS found that women tend to be aware of their husbands' activities.[64] In a survey in Tanzania, women who were asked what actions they had taken predominantly responded that they spoke with their spouses,[65] but separation or divorce has been found elsewhere.[66] The attraction of born-again religions for those concerned about temptation may be widespread; certainly, the proportions who belong to spirit-type churches in which marital fidelity is often a central tenet of faith have been increasing rapidly since the 1970s.[67]

Least well documented in the literature is the role of social networks in the formulation of a navigational chart through the AIDS epidemic, perhaps because, as a recent review of prevention activities notes, the predominant focus in the field of prevention has been on individual behavior.[68] There are some indications, however, of collective responses to the epidemic. To account for Uganda's early decline in HIV, it has been argued that the issue of AIDS had "taken root in social and personal networks in conversations between friends, families, and in communities," so that knowledge of AIDS "would be communicated with advice, or an opinion, and possibly imparted with a sense of trust."[69] More informatively, in focus groups in Uganda in the early 1990s, women "said that they frequently talk about AIDS particularly if a close friend has died of AIDS;" that they talk about "'how to prevent ourselves and others from getting slim.'" "'We just talk about it as though in a conversation. We talk about it on the way to fetch water, when digging ... We ask ourselves why people do not avoid AIDS ...'"[70] Stories of people who were sick with or died from AIDS have stimulated conversations elsewhere. In Zambia people learned about AIDS from "'people discussing and seeing them suffering in the hospital'"; "'hearing many people talking about it and listening to the radio'"; "'neighbors and other people talking about those sick or someone dead'"; or "'seeing a friend suffer from AIDS.'"[71]

Taken together, the evidence of similarities in strategies of prevention and the likely role of social networks suggests that the course of the epidemic may begin to slow in other countries as well. Would the epidemic diminish more quickly if international and national actors had mounted earlier, better, or more interventions to change sexual behavior? The implication of the analysis in this article is that this is unlikely. Money has provided critical resources, such as epidemiological information and accessible condoms, and it could make possible early and effective treatment of the STIs that increase the transmission probabilities of HIV. But I conclude that the fundamental cultural work of coping with AIDS must be done collectively by those whose lives, and whose conceptions of a good life, are threatened. In Malawi, this cultural work is indeed being done and is likely to be effective.

Acknowledgements

I am grateful for comments from Sandra Barnes, Agnes Chimbiri, Georges Reniers, Ann Swidler, and participants in colloquiums at UCLA, Harvard, the California Institute of Technology, Arizona State University, and the University of Pennsylvania. I am also grateful for collaboration with the members of the Malawi Diffusion and Ideational Change Project, and for support from the Rockefeller Foundation; NICHD (R01-HD4173, R01 HD372-276); NIA (AG1236-S3); and the Center for AIDS Research and the Center on the Demography of Aging, both at the University of Pennsylvania.

Notes

[1] Reprinted, with permission, from *Population and Development Review* 30 (December 2004): 673-705.

[2] Ann Swidler, *Talk of Love: How Culture Matters* (Chicago: University of Chicago Press, 2001), 94.

[3] Paul DiMaggio, "Culture and Cognition," *Annual Review of Sociology* 23 (1997): 280. Although demographers have typically shown little interest in either cognition or cultural change, they have long been interested in the major collective event of fertility decline. Much of our research in Malawi has been influenced by the literature on the diffusion of innovations. See Mark R. Montgomery, and John B. Casterline, "Social Influence, Social Learning and New Models of Fertility," in *Fertility in the United States: New Patterns, New Theories, Supplement to Population and Development Review* 22 (1996): 151-75, ed. Ronald D. Lee, Karen A. Foote and John B. Casterline; Thomas W. Valente, *Network Models of the Diffusion of Innovations* (Cresskill, NJ: Hampton Press, 1995); and Alberto Palloni, "Diffusion in Sociological Analysis," in *Diffusion Processes and Fertility Transition*, ed. John B. Casterline (Washington, DC: National Academy Press, 2001), 66-114. Recently, there have been several empirical demonstrations of the role of conversational networks in the adoption of family planning. See Mark R. Montgomery et al., "Social Networks and Contraceptive Dynamics in Southern Ghana," *Population Council Working Paper* No. 153, 2001; John Casterline et al., "Contraceptive Use in Southern Ghana: The Role of Social Networks" (paper presented at the annual meeting of the Population Association of America, Los Angeles, 22-25 March, 2000); and Hans-Peter Kohler, Jere R. Behrman, and Susan C. Watkins, "Social Network Influences and AIDS Risk Perceptions: Tackling the Causality Problem" (paper presented at the annual meeting of the Population Association of America, Atlanta, GA, 9-11 May, 2002). Economists have modeled informational cascades, e.g., Sushil Bikchandani, David Hirshleifer, and Ivo Welch, "A Theory of Fads, Fashions, Custom, and Cultural Change as Informational Cascades," *Journal of Political Economy* 100 (1992): 992-1026, and the way in which social interactions generate social multipliers, e.g., Steven N. Durlauf, and James R. Walker, "Social Interactions and Fertility Transitions," in *Diffusion Processes and Fertility Transition*, ed. John B. Casterline (Washington, DC: National Academy Press, 2001), 115-137.

[4] A third round of the survey was conducted in 2004, but the data are not yet ready for analysis.

[5] See http://www.pop.upenn.edu/networks, and a special collection of Demographic Research at http://www.demographic-research.org.

[6] See e.g., Katharine A. Miller, Eliya Zulu, and Susan C. Watkins, "Husband-wife Survey Responses in Malawi," *Studies in Family Planning* 32 (2001): 161-174; Susan Watkins, Eliya M. Zulu, Hans-Peter Kohler, and Jere R. Behrman, "Demographic Research on HIV/AIDS in Rural Malawi: An Introduction," *Demographic Research* 2003, Special Collection, at http://www.demographic-research.org; Simona Bignami, "Are We Measuring What We Want to Measure? Question Reliability and Individual Consistency in Rural Malawi," *Demographic Research* 2003, Special Collection, at http://www.demographic-research.org.

[7] Katua Munguti et al., "Patterns of Sexual Behaviour in a Rural Population in North-

Western Tanzania," *Social Science & Medicine* 10 (1997): 1533-1561; Brian G. Williams et al., "Changing Patterns of Knowledge, Reported Behaviour and Sexually Transmitted Infections in a South African Gold Mining Community," *AIDS* 17 (2003): 2099-2107; Barbara S. Mensch, Paul C. Hewett, and Annabel S. Erulkar, "The Reporting of Sensitive Behavior by Adolescents: A Methodological Experiment in Kenya," *Demography* 40 (2003): 247-268; Judith M. Stephenson, and Frances Cowan, "Evaluating Interventions for HIV Prevention in Africa," *The Lancet* 361 (2003): 633-634.

[8] Susan Watkins, Hans-Peter Kohler, and Jere R. Behrman, "The Influence of Cross-Gender Network Conversations on Responses to AIDS in Rural Malawi" (paper presented at the annual meeting of the Population Association of America, Boston, 1-3 May 2004); Hans-Peter Kohler, and Stephane Helleringer, "Social Networks, Risk Perception and Changing Attitudes Towards HIV-AIDS: New Evidence from a Longitudinal Study Using Fixe Deffect Estimation" (paper presented at the annual meeting of the Population Association of America, Boston, 1-3 May 2004); Hans-Peter Kohler, Jere R. Behrman, and Susan C. Watkins, "Social Network Influences and AIDS Risk Perceptions"; Kirsten Smith, "Why Are They Worried? Concern about AIDS in Rural Malawi," *Demographic Research* 2003 Special Collection, at http://www.demographic-research.org; Kirsten P. Smith, and Susan C. Watkins, "Perceptions of Risk and Strategies for Prevention: Responses to HIV/AIDS in Rural Malawi," *Social Science & Medicine* 60 (2005): 649-660.

[9] The local ethnographers are young high school graduates (late 20s, early 30s) who went no further in school. There is widespread underemployment of high school graduates in Malawi. Most seek jobs in the cities, but many are unsuccessful and return to their villages. Their homes are in or near villages covered by our survey; and, like the other village residents, they rely primarily on subsistence agriculture supplemented by casual labor or small-scale retail. At the beginning of the journal project, in 1999, we selected the best six of those who had worked for the project both as survey interviewers in 1998 and again as qualitative interviewers in 1999. Two of these are female, the others male. Conversations are typically gender-specific, which means that, regrettably, the journals provide more insight into the conversations of men than of women. There are, however, mixed-gender conversations, and sometimes the females overheard male conversations and vice versa. Of these six journalists, four (one female, three male) were the most active (one male began higher schooling in a city, and one female married and moved out of the area). These four live in different villages, but knew each other by name before they began working as survey interviewers for our project. Subsequently, their interaction increased, but is sporadic: for example, they do not appear to attend the same funerals.

At various points in the journal project we offered others a chance to write journals, but with the exception of one woman who joined the project in 2004, none of those proved satisfactory: they either tried to imitate a survey format, or they wrote vague paragraphs about local customs, or they dropped out, apparently because writing down their recollections was not as profitable or congenial an activity as other opportunities. More detail is available at http://www.pop.upenn.edu/Social_Networks/qualitative/ malawi. As of September 2004, we have approximately 300 journals, each about 7,500 words, covering the period of five years from late 1999 to the present. Some journalists contributed only a few journals a year, others as many as 75 a year. Their journal activities probably take the better part of two or three days a week. The journalists sometimes note how long the conversation lasted and how long it took them to write the journal: roughly, it appears that about two hours of conversation took about six to eight hours to write. Some journals consist of one long conversation, which may extend to two journals; others are a series of briefer conversations. Fewer journals were written between 1999 and 2001, more subsequently. We do not think that this was due to an increase in conversations about AIDS; rather, the increase in grain prices following poor crops in 2001 and a famine in 2002 led the journalists to go more often to places such as the trading center where they could expect more conversational activity. The increase in productivity does not appear to be accompanied by a decrease in quality. In what follows, excerpts from journals are identified by a pseudonym for the journalist and the year the journal was written. All names of individuals and local places have been changed as well.

[10]Miller McPherson, Lynn Smith-Lovin, and James M. Cook, "Birds of a Feather: Homophily in Social Networks," *Annual Review of Sociology* 27 (2001): 415-444; Ina Warriner and Susan Cotts Watkins, "How Do We Know We Need to Control for Selectivity?," *Demographic Research* 2003 Special Collection, http://www.demographic-research.org.

[11]Amy Kaler, "'My Girlfriends Could Fill a Yanu-Yanu Bus': Rural Malawian Men's Beliefs about Their Own Serostatus," *Demographic Research, 2003 Special Collection,* http://www.demographic-research.org.

[12]World Bank, "World Development Indicators Database," 2002, at http://www.worldbank.org/data/databytopic/GNPPC.pdf.

[13]Wiseman C. Chirwa, "Sexually Transmitted Diseases in Colonial Malawi," in *Histories of Sexually Transmitted Diseases and HIV/AIDS in Sub-Saharan Africa,* ed. Philip W. Setel, Milton Lewis, and Maryinez Lyons (Westport, CT: Greenwood Press, 1999), 143-66; Jane Rowley, and Seth Berkley, "Sexually Transmitted Diseases," in *Dimensions of Sex and Reproduction,* vol. III, ed. Christopher J. L. Murray and Alan D. Lopez (Boston, MA: Harvard School of Public Health, 1998), 19-109.

[14]On sexually transmitted infections in the colonial period, see Chirwa, "Sexually Transmitted Diseases in Colonial Malawi." Elderly people in one of our survey sites were asked to compare health conditions in their younger days and today; Amy Kaler generously made available the transcripts of these interviews. The elderly starkly contrasted the fatality of AIDS with the STIs of their youth. Although initially there was no cure for the STIs, eventually "the Europeans brought medicine, so they could be easily cured."

[15]Paula Tavrow, *Family Planning Knowledge, Attitudes and Practices: Machinga District, 1993,* (Machinga District Health Office and GTZ/Liwonde, Zomba: Centre for Social Research, University of Malawi, 1994).

[16]See Table 21 in Tavrow, *Family Planning Knowledge, Attitudes and Practices.* Under President Banda, epidemiological information and prevention prescriptions were disseminated through the press, and these were probably supplemented by information spread through social networks. Although the dissemination of information on AIDS from international agencies to national governments in Africa began in the mid-1980s, a review of press coverage between 1985 and 1991 showed that the government-controlled press in Malawi published little on the epidemic, and what there was consisted primarily of epidemiological information and reports of AIDS elsewhere; not until 1993 were estimates of HIV prevalence in Malawi published. See Anne-Marie Wangel, "AIDS in Malawi – A Case Study: A Conspiracy of Silence?" (dissertation for Master of Science in Pub-

lic Health in Developing Countries, London School of Hygiene and Tropical Medicine, 1995). Nonetheless, information probably spread informally. For example, between 1988 and 1992 about 13,000 Malawian migrant mine workers were repatriated from South Africa on the grounds that their serotesting showed that 200 of them were HIV positive. See Wiseman C. Chirwa, "Aliens and AIDS in Southern Africa: The Malawi-South Africa Debate," *African Affairs* 97 (1998): 53-79. Because remittances from migrant mine workers had been important to rural families since colonial times, it is likely that many in the rural villages would have discussed AIDS in the context of the repatriation.

[17] Lisa Garbus, *HIV/AIDS in Malawi* (San Francisco, CA: AIDS Policy Research Center, AIDS Research Institute, University of California San Francisco, 1993), 68.

[18] UNAIDS, "Epidemiological Fact Sheet," Malawi, 2004 update, at http://www.who.int/GlobalAtlas/PDFFactory/HIV/EFS_PDFs/EFS2004_MW.pdf (accessed 4 November 2004.)

[19] Geoff P. Garnett, Nicholas C. Grassley, and Simon Gregson, "AIDS: The Makings of a Development Disaster?," *Journal of International Development* 13 (2001): 391-392.

[20] R. H. L'Herminez, M. A. G. Hofts, and W. N. Chiwaya, "AIDS in Mangochi District: Clinical Presentation," *Malawi Medical Journal* 8 (1992): 113-117.

[21] Heanry V. Doctor, "Insights From Census and Longitudinal Data on Adult Mortality in Malawi" (Ph.D. dissertation, Graduate Group in Demography, University of Pennsylvania, 2002).

[22] In 2001 a project team member, Patrick Gerland, informally asked village leaders in one of our sites when the first death from AIDS of a person they knew had occurred. Informants variously recalled deaths in 1992, 1994, and 1997. Focus groups conducted in an urban hospital in Malawi give approximately the same dating: "All the men felt that they would not be surprised if they were told that they were HIV positive. This was largely because they were all promiscuous until the 1990s when they started seeing their friends suffering and dying of AIDS." See Thomas J. Bisika, *Behavioral Component of the Preparatory AIDS Vaccine Evaluation (PAVE) Studies* (Centre for Social Research, University of Malawi, in collaboration with Johns Hopkins University, 1995), 8-9.

[23] Angela Chimwaza and Susan C. Watkins, "Giving Care to People with Symptoms of AIDS in Rural Sub-Saharan Africa," *AIDS Care* 16 (2004): 795-807.

[24] Matthew Rabin, "Psychology and Economics," *Journal of Economic Literature* 36 (1998):11-46, citing Daniel Kahneman and Amos Tversky, "On the Psychology of Prediction," *Psychology Review* 80 (1973): 237-251.

[25] Kaler, "'My Girlfriends Could Fill a Yanu-Yanu Bus.'"

[26] Deborah Helitzer-Allen, *An Investigation of Community-Based Communication Networks of Adolescent Girls in Rural Malawi for HIV/STD Prevention Messages*, Research Report Series No. 4 (Washington, DC: International Center for Research on Women, 1994); Claire Hickey, *Factors Explaining Observed Patterns of Sexual Behavior. Phase 2-Longitudinal Study, Final Report* (Zomba: Centre for Social Research, University of Malawi, 1999). Helitzer-Allen conducted focus groups and interviews with adolescent females in Malawi, who said they discussed their sexual experiences with friends. In a focus group of girls aged 9 to 12 years, girls who had had sex reported having talked with their friends about the sexual encounter, "especially when girls are in their multitudes at the river or when going or coming from school" (p. 62). In a focus group of 13-15-year old girls, one said, "I found three girls at the open well telling each other how they feel

when doing sex. One was telling her friends that her first time to do sex she felt very painful but now she feels OK and she does enjoy it" (ibid.). In her study in Mchinji, one of our research sites, Hickey produced similar findings. I am grateful to her for making available to me the texts of the interviews, which were summarized rather than tape recorded and transcribed. In the interviews, women said they often discussed sex, both because it was enjoyable to do and because they could learn from the experiences of others. In the transcript of one of Hickey's interviews, the respondent was reported to have said, "In their discussion they teach one another on how to take care of their husband so that he should be satisfied with them. This can avoid their husbands to go for other women. There are situations where her friends consult for her assistance. There might be a situation whereby their husband is not having sex with them and they get worried why this is so." Another respondent said, "She discusses sexual matters and sexuality with others. She engages in such discussions almost everyday. She discusses this with her friends from the village and also her husband. She feels she does the right thing when she discusses sex because she needs to know since she is newly married and lacks experience while her friends have wide experience in sexual matters and sexuality. She says what she does is to discuss sexual matters with her female friends during daytime and at night rediscuss the same issues with her husband since she enjoys this so much."

[27] The anthropologist J. A. Barnes, who worked in Malawi in the 1950s, wrote that at the time it was assumed that if a husband was away for as much as a month the wife might seek another sexual partner (J. A. Barnes, *Marriage in a Changing Society: A Study in Structural Change Among the Fort Jameson Ngoni*, New York: Oxford University Press, 1951). Claire Hickey's interviews cited previously asked about the frequency of sex within marriage. Her interviews show that frequencies of four times per week are considered normal and desirable, although this level is often reduced, for example in the late stages of pregnancy and the postpartum period or by illness or travel (Hickey, *Factors Explaining Observed Patterns of Sexual Behavior*).

[28] Kaler, "'My Girlfriends Could Fill a Yanu-Yanu Bus'"

[29] Linda Tawfik, "Soap, Sweetness, and Revenge: Patterns of Sexual Onset and Partnerships Amidst AIDS in Rural Southern Malawi" (Ph.D. dissertation, Bloomberg School of Public Health, Johns Hopkins University, Baltimore, MD, 2003); Linda Tawfik and Susan C. Watkins, "Sex in Geneva, Sex in Lilongwe and Sex in Balaka" (paper presented at the annual meeting of the Population Association of America, 1-3 May, 2003).

[30] Our survey included several questions from the Malawi Demographic and Health Surveys in order to evaluate the national representativeness of our sample.

[31] United Nations, *HIV/AIDS Awareness and Behavior* (New York: Population Division, Department of Economic and Social Affairs, 2002).

[32] See also Smith, and Watkins, "Perceptions of Risk and Strategies for Prevention."

[33] Ronald H. Gray et al., "Probability of HIV-1 Transmission per Coital Act in Monogamous, Heterosexual, HIV-1 Discordant Couples in Rakai, Uganda," *The Lancet* 357 (2001): 1149-1153; Rowley and Berkley, "Sexually Transmitted Diseases."

[34] Chiweni Chimbwete and Susan C. Watkins, "Repentance and Hope among Christians and Muslims in Rural Malawi," *Religion in Malawi* 11 (2004): 1-13; David B. Barrett, George T. Kurian, and Todd M. Johnson, *World Christian Encyclopedia*, 2nd ed., vol. 1 (New York: Oxford University Press, 2001); R. A. Van Dijk, "Young Puritan preachers in post-independence Malawi," *Africa* 62 (1992): 159-181.

[35] Eliya M. Zulu and Gloria Chepngeno, "Spousal Communication and Management of HIV/AIDS Risk in Rural Malawi," *Demographic Research* Special Collection, 2003, http://www.demographicresearch.org.

[36] Enid Schatz, "Numbers and Narratives: Making Sense of Gender and Context in Rural Malawi" (Ph.D. dissertation, University of Pennsylvania, 2002); Enid Schatz, "Measuring or Misrepresenting: Assessing Women's Situation in Rural Malawi," *Demographic Research* Special Collection, 2003, http://www.demographic-research.org; Tawfik, "Soap, Sweetness, and Revenge;" Tawfik and Watkins, "Sex in Geneva, Sex in Lilongwe and Sex in Balaka."

[37] Tawfik and Watkins, "Sex in Geneva, Sex in Lilongwe and Sex in Balaka."

[38] Fidelity is particularly central in the preaching of the spirit-type denominations (e.g., Pentecostal, Evangelical) that have been increasingly attractive to people in Malawi and elsewhere, and to which approximately 20 percent of our sample respondents belong. See Ruth Marshall, "Power in the Name of Jesus," *Review of African Political Economy* 52 (1991): 21-37; Van Dijk, "Young Puritan Preachers in Post-Independence Malawi."

[39] Simon Gregson, Tom Zhuwau, Roy M. Anderson, and Stephen K. Chandiwana, "Apostles and Zionists: The Influence of Religion on Demographic Change in Rural Zimbabwe," *Population Studies* 53 (1999): 179-193.

[40] Claire Noël, "A Question of Faith: Membership in a Spirit-Type Church Associated with Distinct Behavior and Attitudes Regarding the HIV/AIDS Epidemic in Rural Malawi?" (unpublished paper, 2003).

[41] Chimbwete and Watkins, "Repentance and Hope Among Christians and Muslims in Rural Malawi."; Van Dijk, "Young Puritan Preachers in Post-Independence Malawi."

[42] Amy Kaler, "AIDS-Talk in Everyday Life: HIV/AIDS in Men's Informal Conversations in Rural Malawi," *Social Science and Medicine* 59 (2004): 285-298.

[43] Adam Ashforth, "Weighing Manhood in Soweto," *CODESRIA Bulletin* 3 & 4 (1999): 51-58.

[44] Amy Kaler, "The Moral Lens of Population Control: Condoms and Controversies in Southern Malawi," *Studies in Family Planning* 35 (2004): 105-115.

[45] For Kenya, see Sarah Thomsen et al., "Fifty Ways to Leave Your Rubber: How Men in Mombasa Rationalize Unsafe Sex" (paper presented at the annual meeting of the Population Association of America, Minneapolis, MN, 1-3 May, 2003); for Zambia, see Virginia Bond and Paul Dover, "Men, Women and the Trouble with Condoms: Problems Associated with Condom Use by Migrant Workers in Rural Zambia," *Health Transition Review* 7 (Suppl, 1997): 377-391; and for eight countries in sub-Saharan Africa, see Sohail Agha et al., *Reasons for Non-Use of Condoms in Eight Countries in Sub-Saharan Africa*. Working Paper No 49 (Washington, DC: PSI, Research Division, 2002).

[46] Smith and Watkins, "Perceptions of Risk and Strategies for Prevention." For similar results from an analysis of Malawi Demographic and Health Survey data, see Agnes Chimbiri, "The Condom Is an 'Intruder in Marriage': Evidence from Rural Malawi," *Social Science & Medicine* 64 (2003): 1102-1115.

[47] Population Services International, Unpublished tables of condom sales by year, 2001; Laura Porter et al., "HIV Status and Union Dissolution in Sub-Saharan Africa: The Case of Rakai, Uganda," *Demography* 41 (2004): 465-482. Since Condoms from Population Services International are sold rather than distributed free (as is the case in the government clinics), it is likely that the people who buy them intend to use them.

[48] Chimbiri, "The Condom Is an 'Intruder in Marriage'."

[49] Schatz, "Numbers and Narratives."

[50] Shelley Clark, "Suspicion, Infidelity and HIV Among Married Couples in Malawi" (paper presented at the annual meeting of the Population Association of America, Minneapolis, MN, 1-3 May, 2003).

[51] Smith and Watkins, "Perceptions of Risk and Strategies for Prevention."

[52] Zulu and Chepngeno, "Spousal Communication and Management of HIV/AIDS Risk in Rural Malawi."

[53] Georges Reniers, "Divorce in rural Malawi," *Demographic Research* Special Collection, 2003, at http://www.demographic-research.org. Here, a life-table analysis of the marital histories collected by our survey in 2001 showed that approximately 50 percent of all first marriages ended in divorce within 30 years, and of these most ended within 15 years. It is not possible to say whether divorce rates increased when villagers perceived that AIDS was a threat to themselves. Although divorce has not been advised by prevention programs, it is a strategy consistent with longstanding practice: the anthropologist Clyde Mitchell, who conducted fieldwork in the late 1940s and early 1950s in an area that is part of our research site, found what he considered a high rate of divorce. See J. C. Mitchell, "The Yao of Southern Nyasaland," in *Seven Tribes of Central Africa*, 2nd ed., ed. Elizabeth Colson and Max Gluckman (Manchester, England: Manchester University Press, 1968), 292-351.

[54] Barnes, *Marriage in a Changing Society*.

[55] Pranitha Maharaj, and John Cleland, "Condom Use Within Marital and Cohabiting Partnerships," *Studies in Family Planning* 35 (2004): 116-124.

[56] Michael Bracher, Gigi Santow, and Susan C. Watkins, "'Moving' and Marrying: Modelling HIV Infection among Newly-Weds in Malawi," *Demographic Research* Special Collection, 2003, http://www.demographic-research.org.

[57] Michael Bracher, Gigi Santow, and Susan C. Watkins, "A Microsimulation Study of the Effects of Divorce and Remarriage on Lifetime Risk of HIV/AIDS in Rural Malawi" (paper presented at the annual meeting of the Population Association of America, Minneapolis, MN, 1-3 May, 2003).

[58] United Nations, *HIV/AIDS Awareness and Behavior*.

[59] Philip Setel, Milton Lewis, and Maryinez Lyons, eds., *Histories of Sexually Transmitted Diseases and HIV/AIDS in Sub-Saharan Africa* (Westport, CT: Greenwood Press, 1999).

[60] For Uganda, see Rebecca E. Bunnell, "Promoting or Paralyzing Behavior Change: Understanding Gender and High Levels of Perceived Risk of HIV Infection in Southwestern Uganda" (Ph.D. dissertation, Harvard University, 1996). For Zimbabwe, see Gregson, Zhuwau, Anderson, and Chandiwana, "The Early Socio-Demographic Impact of the HIV-1 Epidemic in Rural Zimbabwe."

[61] For Zambia, see Bond and Dover, "Men, Women and the Trouble with Condoms." For South Africa, see Christine A. Varga, "The Condom Conundrum: Barriers to Condom Use among Commercial Sex Workers in Durban, South Africa," *African Journal of Reproductive Health* 1 (1997): 74-88, and Catherine Campbell, *'Letting Them Die': Why HIV/AIDS Prevention Programmes Fail* (Bloomington: Indiana University Press, 2003). For Uganda, see Tony Barnett, and Piers Blaikie, *AIDS in Africa: Its Present and Future Impact* (New York: Guilford Press, 1992).

[62] Gregson, Zhuwau, Anderson, and Chandiwana, "The Early Socio-Demographic Impact of the HIV-1 Epidemic in Rural Zimbabwe," 346. See also, for South Africa, Campbell, *'Letting Them Die.'*

[63] For Kenya, see C. Nzioka, "Lay Perceptions of Risk of HIV Infection and the Social Construction of Safer Sex: Some Experiences from Kenya," *AIDS CARE* 8 (1996): 565-579. For Rwanda, see Anne-Emmanuèle Calvès, *1998 Rwanda Sexual Behavior and Condom Use Survey; First Report* (Washington, DC: PSI: Social Marketing and Communications for Health, n.d.). For Tanzania, see Robert Pool, Mary Maswe, J. T. Boerma, and Soori Nnko, "The Price of Promiscuity: Why Urban Males in Tanzania Are Changing Their Sexual Behaviour," *Health Transition Review* 6 (1996): 203-221. For Uganda, see Bunnell, "Promoting or Paralyzing Behavior Change." For South Africa, see Campbell, *'Letting Them Die.'*

[64] Barney Cohen, and James E. Trussell, *Preventing and Mitigating AIDS in Sub-Saharan Africa: Research and Data Priorities for the Social and Behavioral Sciences* (Washington, DC: National Research Council, 1996).

[65] Gregson, Zhuwau, Anderson, and Chandiwana, "The Early Socio-Demographic Impact of the HIV-1 Epidemic in Rural Zimbabwe."

[66] For Uganda, see Bunnell, "Promoting or Paralyzing Behavior Change;" and Porter et al., "HIV Status and Union Dissolution in Sub-Saharan Africa."

[67] Barrett, Kurian, and Johnson, *World Christian Encyclopedia.*

[68] Jane T. Bertrand, "Diffusion of innovations and HIV/AIDS," *Journal of Health Communication* 9 (2004): 113-121.

[69] Daniel Low-Beer, and Rand Stoneburner, "Uganda and the Challenge of AIDS," in *The Political Economy of AIDS in Africa*, ed. Nana K. Poku and Alan Whiteside (Aldershot: Ashgate Publishing, 2004), 165-190.

[70] Magid Kagimu et al., "Evaluation of the Effectiveness of AIDS Health Education Interventions in the Muslim Community in Uganda," *AIDS Education and Prevention* 10 (1998): 222.

[71] Ann Sikwibele, Caroline Shonga, and Carolyn Baylies, "AIDS in Kapulanga, Mongu: Poverty, Neglect and Gendered Patterns of Blame," in *AIDS, Sexuality and Gender in Africa: Collective Strategies and Struggles in Tanzania and Zambia*, ed. Carolyn Baylies and Janet Bujra (London: Routledge, 2000), 68.

CHAPTER 5

HIV/AIDS in Africa: No More Slogans

EVELYNE SHUSTER

In the postmodern world of globalization, the Internet, and TV images, it
is impossible to ignore how most people on our planet live and die. AIDS
is now the leading cause of death worldwide for people aged 15 to 50, two-
thirds of which in sub-Saharan Africa.[1] In the 25 years since the first case of
AIDS was discovered, 60 million people have been infected, 25 million have
suffered agonizing and horrendous deaths, and millions of children have
been orphaned. Despite politically charged efforts to contain the epidemic,
an estimated five million people a year continue to be infected. Statistics
of this magnitude as well as death images tend to overwhelm rather than
inspire human resolve, and have produced more slogans and nonbinding
declarations than concrete, realistic and sustainable solutions.

There is nothing hopeful about the AIDS epidemic. As the world marks
the 25th anniversary of the detection of HIV, United Nations Secretary
General Kofi Annan gloomily declares that the world is losing the battle,
and "the epidemic continues to outpace us."[2] Nicholas Kristof, *New York
Times* reporter and activist agrees, saying that "this has been a sad chapter
in the history of humanity, a quarter century of self-delusion, dithering and
failure at every level."[3] Efforts to stem the epidemic have chronically fallen
short despite promises by world leaders (and others) to directly engage in
AIDS awareness, education, prevention, and treatment. Time and again,
promises and plans have been negotiated and renegotiated between periods
of bickering and calls for unity.[4] The United States, for example, has
repeatedly pledged to give a larger share of its gross national product (GNP)
but, year after year, has fallen short of its 0.7% goal. Its current level of
aid is a paltry 0.15% of GNP. The G8 nations have vowed to double their
annual aid to Africa, i.e. an increase of 25 billion dollars a year by 2010,

when in fact they needed to commit 50 billion to reflect the target of 0.7% of GNP.[5] A pledge by the World Health Organization (WHO) to treat an additional three million AIDS patients in poor countries by the end of 2005 (the 3 by 5 program) failed to achieve its goal by more than one million.[6] As it was bluntly put, "2005 is likely to be remembered more for the 3 million deaths and almost five million new infections it heralded than for the 300,000 lives saved through treatment."[7]

Yet, the new millennium began with high expectations. Looking at the bright side, myriad declarations, programs, proposals, development goals have been presented to address the epidemic in Africa. For example, the United Nations (UN) Millennium Declaration was acclaimed with great fanfare and signed by almost all member states, directly leading to the adoption of the Millennium Development Goals (MDGs). These goals included nine specific objectives to be realized by 2015, specifically to eliminate extreme poverty, achieve universal primary education, promote gender equality, reduce child and maternal mortality, combat HIV/AIDS, malaria, and other diseases, ensure environmental sustainability, and develop a global partnership for development.

Newly formed non-governmental organizations (NGOs) like Global AIDS Alliance (GAA), actively offered to hasten the end of global AIDS, and identified three major goals: 1) universal access to safe, effective and affordable treatment; 2) a comprehensive, science-based HIV prevention strategy; and 3) a comprehensive social safety net for orphans and vulnerable children. GAA also called for debt cancellation for extremely poor countries (people living with less than one dollar per day) so that they can apply these funds to AIDS education, prevention and treatment. Most recently, GAA has suggested a debt conversion program that could generate additional resources for the newly created UN Global Fund to fight AIDS, tuberculosis and malaria.[8]

Physicians for Human Rights (PHR) urgently called for rich nations to "keep their promises"[9] – assist poor nations with financial, educational, and technical support; increase access to drugs and vaccines; and help them develop their own public health, social, educational, and treatment programs. However, because of extremely difficult working conditions, a great number of nurses and physicians have left African countries. PHR has strongly denounced the depletion of health professionals, which aggravates an already tenuous healthcare work force, leading to an alarming situation.

The shortage of responsible health professionals has been particularly vexing once promises to increase foreign aid have materialized. The United States, with 5 percent of the world's population, now employs more than 11 percent of the globe's physicians, and its demand is growing. For example, the 2005 Global War on Terror, and Tsunami Relief Act includes approval for more than 50,000 new visas for nurses and their families. PHR has called for developed nations "to meet their own health care need without reducing the capacity of developing countries," and insists that rich nations realize their obligations following the World Health Assembly Resolution (57/19), International Migration of Health Personnel. As one commentator accurately put it, "it seems like a cruel joke to play: providing funds for AIDS care but simultaneously taking away the nurses who can give that care."[10]

The lack of political will, misinformation by African leaders about the extent of the epidemic in their own countries, and failure to enforce anti discrimination laws to protect AIDS patients have also been denounced.[11] As it turns out, showing a willingness to assist nations in need, or even actually offering to help directly manage the AIDS crisis has not been sufficient to create good governance and partnership. To built trusted partnerships to overcome mistrust between nations, particularly when these are former colonies, is especially challenging.[12] Perhaps more than economic disparity, a major obstacle to trusting relationships between nations has been the legacy of colonialism. In other words, what could have been realized economically has not been achieved because of the political and emotional fall out of such legacy. As a result of all of these the AIDS epidemic seems intrinsically and fundamentally unmanageable.

The millennium also began with a renewed emphasis on human rights, specifically the right to health. For example, human rights activist and first president of South Africa, Nelson Mandela, challenged the world at the 2000 international AIDS conference in Durban, South Africa, and his challenge remains timely. He exhorted public and private institutions and their leaders to "start on treatment access and make rapid and real progress in achieving treatment goals for all those who need it." Two years after the Durban AIDS Conference, Nelson Mandela again challenged the world – this time at the AIDS conference in Barcelona – in these words: "No one can stand by and watch while children suffer. As adults we have a collective and individual responsibility and obligation to care for and support people living with HIV/AIDS, whoever and wherever they are." Mandela called on all individuals to know their HIV status, and to demand it "as a right to know." Describing AIDS as "a war against humanity," Mandela summoned "political and business leaders, including union, religious, traditional, and NGOs leaders, to show strong leadership as a requisite for an effective response to the 'war against AIDS.'"[13]

Mandela was right to call for universal mobilization. He thereby chose a philosophy of engagement over a philosophy of indifference or a "bystander" ethics. But exactly what are nations obligated to do, and why? How should they do it? I will address these questions, using four different models. Each model has been widely advocated by one leader or another as a way to engage and be engaged in the AIDS pandemic. These four models include the humanitarian, military, commercial, and human rights models. I will make some observations about their applicability in postcolonial Africa, and conclude by suggesting realistic steps that can be taken today to respond to the growing HIV/AIDS pandemic in sub-Saharan Africa.

The Humanitarian Model

Humanitarian values are perhaps best illustrated in our communal responses to help victims of natural or man-made disasters, like tsunamis, hurricanes, floods, droughts, earthquakes, famines, and wars. Humanitarian assistance usually transcends political affiliation and is independent of governmental politics as, for example, relief provided during the 2005 Kashmir earthquake. Natural disasters appear to most of us as undeserved and their victims blameless. These "acts of God" produce almost instant identification, and call for (and receive) universal assistance as the "right" thing to do: humans ought to help their fellow humans in time of need and despair.

Rhetoric often runs high. President George Bush in his January 2001 inaugural address said, "Where there is suffering, there is duty. I pledge our nation to a goal: when we see that wounded traveler on the road to Jericho, we will not pass to the other side."[14] And former president Bill Clinton declared at the opening of the National Summit on Africa, in February 2000: "We can choose to be indifferent or we can make a difference." Echoing earlier statements, Clinton continued:

> The AIDS pandemic is primarily a humanitarian issue. Everybody

counts, everybody has a role to play, and everybody deserves a chance. And we all do better when we help each other. That is a rule we ought to follow with Africa, and we can make it clear to our African partners that we consider AIDS not just their burden but ours as well.

President Clinton was expressing his humanitarian view that "the philosophy and principles by which we ought to act are relatively simple, and based on mutual assistance and respect," – solidarity and human dignity.[15]

To provide humanitarian assistance to victims of natural or man-made disasters is purely a voluntary and charitable act. It constitutes what 18th century German philosopher Immanuel Kant called an "imperfect duty" or "duty of virtue." By this Kant meant that humanitarian acts cannot be forced on people. Not to be charitable is not an offense punishable by law. It is, however, an indication of "moral unworthiness." Imperfect duty contrasts with "perfect duty" or "strict duty" (of right). Acts of perfect duty are obligatory and, when transgressed or violated, are legally punishable. Humanitarian acts are generally carried out by neutral and non-confrontational organizations, like the International Committee of the Red Cross, Oxfam, and religious missionary groups. In time of natural disasters which, unlike an epidemic, have generally a brief time frame, humanitarian organizations request public donations for food, money or supply for immediate relief. Usually, countries and individuals around the world respond positively and generously to humanitarian calls for help because they are able to directly identify with the victims who could just as easily have been them or their relatives.

A bystander ethics or an ethics of indifference or non-interference is simply not acceptable. Nobel Laureate Elie Wiesel would agree. He has asked,

> How could it [the Holocaust] have happened? Some bystanders sought to exploit the situation of the Jews for personal gain, but most people simply stood by, neither collaborating nor coming to the aid of the victims. This passivity amounted to acquiescence, and the planners and executors of the Final Solution counted on bystanders not to intervene in the process of genocide.[16]

Philosopher Jonathan Glover also has rejected a bystander ethics, stating that "any ethical theory that either justifies this tragedy [the Holocaust] or gives no help in avoiding it, is fundamentally inadequate."[17] South

African Justice Edwin Cameron brought this point home when he declared at the opening session of the Durban, AIDS conference, "No more than Germans during the Nazi era, no more than white South Africans during Apartheid can we say we bear no responsibility for more than thirty million people in resources poor countries who face death from AIDS unless medical care and treatment is made accessible to them."[18]

Responsibility and compassion also run high in George W. Bush's 2001 inaugural address. He rhetorically asked the American people "to seek a common good beyond your comfort; to defend needed reforms against easy attacks; to serve your nation, beginning with your neighbor." He continued, "I ask you to be citizens. Citizens, not spectators; citizens not subjects; responsible citizens, building communities of service and a nation of character."[19] By this, he meant that passivity in the face of evil is unacceptable. People cannot morally be passive spectators to human devastation. All of these grand pronouncements, however, have failed to make a significant difference in President Bush's engagement (and ours) in dealing with AIDS in poor countries. We could not sufficiently identify with HIV/AIDS African patients in order to assist those in need. We are witnessing the waste of lives because of the world's indifference to poverty, disease, inequality and global discrimination. Whether it has ever been acceptable for rich nations to stand by and watch people die from lack of treatment because they cannot afford to pay for it is highly problematic. But rich nations have continued to act as if it were, holding no illusions that they could (or should?) overcome Africa's internal conflicts, political turmoil, psychosocial problems and economic difficulties. Nor do rich nations seem to hold out much hope of ever being able to help transform African nations, either through financial support or economic growth. The perception has been that there are too many inadequacies, too much corruption and incompetence.

Though it may have seemed "natural" to look at the HIV/AIDS epidemic in Africa from a humanitarian and charitable perspective, the reality is that it has not been sufficient, and may even have been damaging to the urgency of what is needed to seriously address the epidemic. Indeed, by framing HIV/AIDS more as a "soft" (humanitarian and charitable) issue, rather than as a "hard" (e.g., national security or economic stability) concern, the humanitarian model has contributed to disengage those who could have been committed to help, because it presented the epidemic as a problem that requires charitable solutions, not strong and enduring commitments. And thus this model has been ineffective and inadequate to make any difference in the lives of those who suffer from the disease. Images of people with AIDS, portrayed again and again over the past two decades, have caused us to become accustomed to them and to ultimately treat people with AIDS "either with pity or with indifference."[20]

The Military Model

The continued ineffectiveness of the humanitarian model in dealing with the AIDS pandemic finally prompted both the Clinton and Bush administrations to reframe HIV/AIDS as a national security crisis (a "hard" issue), and to adopt a military model in an effort to mobilize support to fight a sustained "war on AIDS." President Bill Clinton, for example, declared AIDS a "threat to security,"[21] a qualification he had hoped would increase the level of funding in the efforts against AIDS, mainly in Africa. He elevated AIDS research and work to the federal level, to include the National Security Council and the Department of Defense, the first occasion in US history where a global health issue was raised to this status. His Vice-President, Al Gore, addressed the United Nations Security Council, saying that AIDS was not just a humanitarian issue, it threatened not just individual citizens, but the very core of institutions that defined the character of a society. Jus like war, the disease ruins economies, undermines the very survival of societies, destabilizes governments, and causes international insecurity. Gore called for a total mobilization of the nations of the world, in these terms: "AIDS is a global aggressor that must be defeated; it is one of the most devastating threats to confront the world community. Many have called the battle against it a sacred crusade." Gore ended his speech solemnly declaring, "May God bless all who have suffered from this disease. May God bless the united effort of our united nations to end it – soon and forever."[22] By adopting such a stance, Gore was hoping to stimulate a "collective unconscious association of a battle of good against evil, in which any means justify the ends."[23] Under George Bush, his Secretary of State, Colin Powell, adopted the military model even more enthusiastically, declaring

> No war on the face of the world is more destructive than the AIDS pandemic. I am a soldier, but I know of no enemy in war more insidious or vicious than AIDS, an enemy that poses a clear and present

danger to the world. From now on, the world's response to the disease must be no less comprehensive and no less swift that the pandemic itself. AIDS is the world's most dangerous weapon of mass destruction.[24]

The use of war (or military) metaphors has been common in political circles because, as a former CIA analyst put it, war metaphors drive a tendency for absolute solutions. President Bush, for example, prefers to call himself "Commander-in-Chief," perhaps because in this role, unlike in his democratic role as president, he can simply "command" action.[25] Although he usually speaks in human rights terms, even Nelson Mandela, as above noted, has characterized AIDS as "a war against humanity," which "requires mobilization of an entire population." The U.N. General Assembly has likewise noted that the AIDS pandemic impacts on world peace, stability and security, and held a special session on the disease. In the same vein, the CIA's report, *The Global Infectious Disease Threat and its Implication for the United States*, characterizes AIDS as a "threat to our national interest."[26]

War metaphors that fit the military model also fit the Hobbesian model that validates military involvement for self-interest (rather than for merely empathy-based humanitarian reasons). The reasoning goes like this: if AIDS is a threat to our national security, we must get involved, not because it is what we ought to do (Kantian imperfect duty, humanitarian or moral reasons), but because it is what we *must* do to protect ourselves, our security, and our national interest[27] But in doing what we must to protect ourselves, it is sometimes possible also to fulfill our moral obligations towards our fellow human beings. Although not obvious, these two views are not always mutually exclusive, since by acting in our national interest we can still help people, and sometimes helping people can also be in our national interest. The end results are the same whether the focus is on containing the AIDS epidemic for moral reasons or for self-protection. To put it bluntly, AIDS relief motivated by self-preservation and national security (à la Hobbes) would (or at least should) also end up benefiting people in Africa (humanitarian view). It is at least sometimes the case, as in Bosnia, when we intervened militarily for a humanitarian motive, and the intervention also turned out to be in our own national self-interest.

Humanitarian goals, no matter how compelling, cannot be achieved simply with the power of a gun barrel. Using the military to ensure freedom and promote democracy is inherently contradictory because war creates or exacerbates humanitarian problems, and ultimately the two approaches cannot be easily mixed. For example, after the fall of the Soviet Union, the (first) Bush Administration announced a "New World Order" that included using the military for humanitarian and charitable missions. The first of its kind was the U.S. military mission to provide food to Somalis. Operation Restore Hope began with highly-charged images of starving women and children, and ended with bloody images of a dead American soldier being dragged in the mud behind a truck driven by triumphant warlord-led Somalis. This experience led directly to the failure of the Clinton Administration to even try to prevent the Rwanda genocide, and has undoubtedly impacted on our contemporary inability to intervene militarily and initiate major military missions for humanitarian and human rights reasons in the ongoing Sudanese genocide. Non-governmental human rights organizations, like Médecins Sans Frontières (MSF) rightly insist that "the one essential requirement of providing humanitarian aid in a conflict is to keep military action and humanitarian aid separate."[28] The mixing of roles has a negative impact on both sides of the conflict, the people who need assistance, and those who try to provide it.

Looking at AIDS in Africa as a threat to national security was an attempt to dramatize the severity of the AIDS epidemic and draw the world's attention to mobilize to "win" this "war." As it has turned out, it was difficult for most nations to believe that they were at risk if they did not engage in the war against AIDS. To further declare that the national security of the United States would be seriously threatened by AIDS in Africa was simply not true as a matter of fact, and thus was not a credible strategy to help promote the world's assistance to AIDS sufferers. The real national security threat is terrorism, and there has been no shortage of federal money to wage this war. Our new real war is the "global war against terror" which has taken center stage and has almost immediately caused the United States to further marginalize our obligation to the millions infected with HIV, at least in the context of "war."

The Commerce Model

From the beginning of the epidemic, multinational pharmaceutical corporations have followed the profit principle. These corporations have boldly stated that they do not "give their products away," and that their only obligation is to their stockholders, not to sick people who need their products to survive. *New York Times* reporter, Tina Rosenberg, has observed that this strategy has earned drug companies a public image almost as malignant as that of tobacco companies. She argues that patent laws are malleable. Patients are educable and drug companies vincible. The world's AIDS crisis is solvable.[29] Why then haven't we been able to solve it? Are for-profit pharmaceutical companies the only villains? Do pharmaceutical companies really have an obligation to make their life-saving, life-prolonging products available and affordable to those who need them, or do governments and international agencies like the WHO have a primary obligation to find a way to pay the market price for needed life-saving drugs?

After a quarter of century of HIV/AIDS, we continue to ask these same questions. In 1998, the WHO and six major drug companies, Boehringer-Ingelheim, Bristol Myers Squibb, Glaxo Smith Kline, Hoffmann-La Roche, Merck, and Pfizer, met to discuss drug affordability in Third World countries, one of the most contentious issues for "big pharma." But early on, Pfizer refused to discuss prices for its products, saying, "the price of drugs in the US represents good value, and any discussion of preferential pricing undermines that value in core markets." Pfizer withdrew from the discussion. The five remaining companies announced they would be willing to sell their products at discounted prices, but only under specific, nonnegotiable conditions. These conditions include: unequivocal and ongoing political commitment of recipient countries; responsibility of international agencies to build health care infrastructures, and to monitor patient compliance; delivery of drugs only to efficient, reliable and secure distribution systems to prevent interruption of treatment and diversion of products to black markets; recognition by pharmaceutical companies that drug affordability is an issue in developing countries, only if the UN agencies also recognize that AIDS treatment is a "shared responsibility" of all sectors of society, not only the responsibility of drug manufacturers; and finally, recognition and support for intellectual property rights (drug patent issues).[30]

This last condition meant that countries were expected to renounce using two specific mechanisms, compulsory licensing and parallel importing, which have been permitted by the World Trade Organization under conditions of national emergency. Compulsory licensing gives a country the legal authority to produce drugs without the consent of patent holders (not always a useful power because most resource-poor countries have no drug production capability). Parallel importing permits countries to buy a product at a lower price in other markets, like India, Thailand, or Brazil, and resell the product at home without the consent of the manufacturer. No worldwide agreement was reached. Instead, business deals between drug companies and African governments were made and kept largely secret, particularly concerning price cuts. Each price cut, for each drug in each country was decided separately. Agreements had many restrictive conditions. Peter Piot, the UNAIDS chairman, asked for specific details about price cutting, but four of the five companies refused disclosure. Merck broke rank with the group and teamed up with the Bill and Melinda Gates Foundation to create a $100 million AIDS program in Botswana, a relatively rich, democratic country of 1.7 million people. The goal of the program was to prevent HIV transmission from mother to child, a reasonable goal in a country where 72% of pregnant women are HIV-infected.

The Bristol Myers Squibb (BMS) Program, Secure the Future, also proposed to target women and children with its 5-year, $100 million initiative in 5 countries, namely, South Africa, Botswana, Namibia, Lesotho, and Swaziland. The initiative, which began in 1999, had a dual purpose, to secure the drug company's bottom line, and to show the world that the company cares about people with AIDS. As it turned out, it was difficult for those in charge of the program to seriously focus on both profits and charitable concerns without responding to increasing pressure by the public and NGOs to make their life-saving drug products even more affordable and available to those who needed them to survive.[31]

Secure the Future did not live up to its potential. Its design (particularly the exclusion of men) was flawed, its goals unrealistic, and its plan misguided. Men should have been included because in patriarchal societies men make the rules and decide when, with whom, how, and how often to have sex, and thus drive the epidemic. As one NGO noted angrily in reaction to another program favored by President Bush, the 2001 Global AIDS Program, or ABC Program (Abstinence, Be faithful, and Condom use), "what infects and kills women and their children is less promiscuity than marriage itself. The deadliest thing a woman can do in Africa is to get married." To put it differently, "abstinence is fine for those who are able to abstain, but human beings like to have sex and they should not die because they do have sex."[32] BMS scaled back its ambition, providing free drugs to about 20,000 individuals. The company ultimately changed its focus from treatment to research, investing mainly in American-based charitable institutions (about 77% of the money), a move critical to its financial operation, and its moral or humanitarian reputation in the world.

The commerce model has thus failed because of its exclusive emphasis on maximizing profit, with for-profit corporations paying a mere lip service to humanitarian concerns. The strict control of how and where drugs are distributed and how they are utilized, has made it almost impossible to create an efficient and sustainable drug delivery system, and ensure wide-scale access. As frustration and resentment from all sides grew stronger, the major drug companies decided to return to their original position of protecting their pricing policies, and sponsoring research on new drugs or new uses of existing drugs, rather than concentrating on improving access to currently available HIV/AIDS treatments. As a member of MSF sarcastically put it, "the elephant has given birth to a mouse." On the other hand, it was never the responsibility of the pharmaceutical industry to ensure equitable access to its products. This is the government's role.

The Human Rights Model

The resource availability gap between poor and rich nations has put the enjoyment of health beyond the reach of all but the privileged few. Although there has been much debate over what rich countries can afford in aid relief, there has been much less interest in accepting what they should do to help promote social and economic progress in poor countries. What nations ought to do is defined in the UN Charter, the Universal Declaration of Human Rights (UDHR), and the International Covenant on Economic, Social and Cultural Rights (ICESCR). For example, the 1948 UDHR reads,

> Everyone has the right to a standard of living adequate for the health and well-being of himself and of his family, including food, clothing, housing and medical care and necessary social services, and the right to security in the event of unemployment, sickness, disability, widowhood, old age or other lack of livelihood in circumstances beyond his control. Motherhood and childhood are entitled to special care and assistance. (Article 25)

And the 1966 ICESCR recognizes, among other, the rights to citizens to social security (art. 9); to the widest possible protection and assistance for the family, especially mothers, children and young persons (art. 10); to adequate standard of living (art.11); and to the enjoyment of the highest attainable standard of physical and mental health (art.12). As a corollary to the right to development, the international community has an obligation to assist poor countries to achieve basic human rights, including the right to health.

Human rights organizations, most notably MSF, have argued that NGOs have "a duty to intervene" to prevent human rights abuses, as well as a duty to "break the silence" and denounce those who violate human rights. As former MSF president, Dr. Rony Brauman stated, "we are by nature an organization that is unable to tolerate indifference. We hope that by arousing awareness and a desire to understand, we will also stir up indignation and stimulate action."[33] The "without borderism" philosophy is based on the universality of the human condition and the basic rights of all human beings, including rights to personal security, food, shelter, clean water, medical treatment and health services.[34] As Secretary General Kofi Annan has noted, there is nothing in the UN Charter that precludes the recognition that there are rights beyond borders. UN members must no longer let countries use claims of national sovereignty to cover up flagrant abuses of human rights.

Vigorously applying the human rights model to the AIDS epidemic was first proposed and attempted by Jonathan Mann, founder of the WHO Global Program on AIDS. Mann's vision was to emphasize the "inextricable link between health and human rights." He defended that only by taking human rights seriously it would be possible to effectively contain the epidemic. Respect for human rights – both civil rights (like privacy, the right to be left alone, and nondiscrimination), and economic rights (like the right to health) – is necessary in order to secure the success of programs that address the health conditions of people living with HIV/AIDS.[35] Under basic human rights doctrine, governments that have signed ICESCR have the obligation not just to respect the human rights spelled out there, but to protect and fulfill them as well. Effectively combating HIV/AIDS thus requires taking human rights seriously, including actively resisting and combating stigmatization and discrimination, and promoting gender equality, education, health care, nutrition, and employment. Nelson Mandela powerfully highlighted these very points when he commented about children orphaned by AIDS:

These children will grow up without love and care of their parents, and most of them will be deprived of their basic rights – rights to shelter, food, health and education. Many will be subjected to abuse, exploitation, discrimination, trafficking and loss of inheritance. We have an obligation to provide the proper care and support for these children. Stigma and discrimination inflicted are atrocious and inexcusable. People suffering from AIDS are not killed by the disease itself. They are killed by the stigma surrounding those who have HIV/AIDS.[36]

African governments have a human rights obligation to enforce laws against stigmatization and discrimination of people living with HIV/AIDS. The case of women illustrates just how critical human rights are in dealing effectively with the AIDS epidemic.[37] The social, cultural and economic factors that contribute to gender inequality, oppression, low social status and outright discrimination, have made women and their children most vulnerable to HIV infection. As previously noted, in most economically deprived regions, the lack of empowerment of women makes it impossible for them to negotiate HIV prevention methods, such as condoms, or discuss mutual monogamy. Women are often victims of sexual assault and oppression within their family setting. Once HIV infected, they are rejected by both their families and society, and forced into prostitution and "sexual networking" for food and shelter.[38] As Paul Farmer has (rightly) observed, the threat of HIV/AIDS to women in Africa is less biological than cultural and economic. Farmer is also correct in insisting that the real epidemic the world is facing is not so much an epidemic of HIV/AIDS as an epidemic of inequality.[39] His call for human rights and social justice is further on target, and it takes nothing away from his analysis to note that although the WHO adopted the "health and human rights" framework for its own work, the model so far has not been adequately employed in the real world. The United States, which played a major role in creating the UN and articulating the 1948 Universal Declarations of Human Rights, has indeed – at least since 9/11 – taken a very different role today, that of undermining the international human rights agenda.[40] And, most surprisingly, it has done so by rejecting the very civil and political rights it once accused other nations of failing to adhere to, for example, the Geneva Conventions and the prohibition on torture. It is also unfortunate that in the current supercharged war-on-terror atmosphere, the health and human rights agenda has been all but abandoned, which helps to explain (at least partially) why the human rights model as applied to AIDS has not been very effective.

Failed Models and Postcolonialism

Unless we understand why these four models have not led to successful responses to the HIV/AIDS epidemic, we will not be able to reasonably suggest a way forward. Three factors taken together may explain our past failure. The first involves the way in which facts are presented, often inflated and overstated. For example, it has not been helpful to argue that ignoring Africa's ills may bankrupt our economic future because this is simply not credible. Nor is it credible to argue that non intervention threatens our national or global security. These assertions are a formula for ultimate failure because they are based on pretense.

Similarly, we must be realistic in assessing what exactly rich nations can do to ease the crisis. For example, it is critical to recognize that rich nations cannot bring African living standards (or healthcare standards) to the level of European or American standards. To say otherwise is misleading. It is preferable to argue for a reduction of the economic gap that exists between rich and poor nations, so that progressive (economic) partnerships have a chance to take roots and reasonably develop. In this regard, the Millennium Goal of reducing the number of people currently living on less than a dollar a day is reasonable and significant, even if minimal (although there will always be one billion people who will remain the poorest one billion in the world). It is also unrealistic to argue that rich nations can bring the very fruits of modern science and medicine to countries with fundamentally different levels of economic maturity, even if they are politically similar to ours.

The second factor, as the title of my essay suggests, is a danger of over-promising and using slogans or grand claims to engage developed nations. For example, it is over-promising to claim that we can end poverty, achieve universal education, or treat 3 million people with HIV/AIDS by a certain date. It should be obvious that promises are made to be kept. Promises that are not kept tend to destroy credibility and make us (and Africa) victims of our own device. And if at the beginning we may dream of successfully achieving many desirable goals, at the end there is the nightmarish realization that we pitifully failed, victims of our own hype and illusions. There are limits to how many times we can engage in promoting programs with catchy slogans and promises before all our new programs be greeted with indifference, or worse, cynicism. There are also limits to the number of nonbinding declarations, such as the June 2nd 2006 UN Declaration "to reaffirm commitments made in 2001 that AIDS is far more than a medical issue and should be framed in terms of politics, human rights and economic survival."[41] Understandably, it is difficult to acknowledge that promises were unattainable and thus it is logical for the head of WHO's HIV/AIDS program to qualify its unsuccessful "3 X 5" initiative as "ambitious, and having aspirational target," rather than saying that the "3 X 5" goals were simply over promising, unrealistic and unattainable.[42] We can no longer afford making nonbinding declarations without specific action plans, or moving from one slogan to another without at least acknowledging the factors that led to the failure of the most recent program.[43]

The third factor, and perhaps the most important, is that Africa consists primarily of former colonies. Africans see themselves at risks of further exploitation, particularly when new relationships are formed on the model of previous ones between colonies and colonizers.[44] Overlooking or neglecting this fact undermines any potentially useful partnership, and may fatally harm any potential collaboration and investment. There are those who do not want to be indefinitely responsible for the political and economic shortcomings of developing countries (or former colonies) in which they have invested large sums of money, and there are those who continue to argue that progress and economic benefits require long-term partnerships between countries and sustained collaboration. Both views are partially correct. The former is correct from an economic perspective; the latter from a political and moral perspective. To alleviate Africa's ills can be both economically beneficial and morally and politically rewarding to those willing to invest. We need not (or should not) be bashful or defensive about generating revenues or financial gain when pursuing effective and promising health strategies in poor countries. As French political philosopher, Raymond Aron put it in the context of the French-Algerian relation, "without self-interest – what is there for us – it is unlikely that we would be involved in the first place, and even less committed and engaged in doing what is right for Africa."[45]

Exploitation of the poor may take many forms as illustrated by the controversy ignited by the maternal HIV transmission studies in Africa in the late 1990s. These trials were sponsored by the US National Institutes of Health (NIH) and Centers for Disease Control (CDC), to determine if the so-called 076 AZT regimen, which had proven effective in substantially reducing HIV transmission from mother to child in the United States, would be effective if a much less expensive, lower-dose AZT, was used.[46] Instead of comparing this inexpensive intervention with the proven 076 drug regimen, the study was designed to compare it to a placebo. Peter Lurie and Sidney Wolfe (the Health Research Group arm of Public Citizen, founded by Ralph Nader) accused the US government of sponsoring unethical research studies because the trial did not use the known effective treatment as the control for this experiment.[47] This would have been required had the trial been done in the United States. The use of placebo was also denounced by Marcia Angell, then the executive editor of the *New England Journal of Medicine*, who drew an analogy with the infamous Tuskegee syphilis experiments. Similarly to what happened then, investigators argued that the HIV-infected pregnant women in the AIDS trials would not receive antiretroviral treatment anyway, so they were justified in simply observing what would happen to them and their babies.[48]

Law Professor, Leonard Glantz and his colleagues at Boston University School of Public Health asked whether these trials should have been done at all in countries that have no adequate health services. They noted further that the reason for the research was not medical (a treatment already existed), but economic (to find a cheaper treatment that could be affordable in African countries). They concluded that without a tangible benefit to the population tested, the study was simple exploitation:

> Since the AIDS trials in Africa were done almost exclusively for economic reasons, the sine qua non condition for approval of these trials should have been an actual and realistic economic plan to deliver the tested intervention to the population from which experimental subjects are drawn.[49]

Government regulatory agencies strongly disagreed and continued to defend these clinical trials.[50] The controversy over subject exploitation in the research setting in Africa continues to this day, and has spread to Southeast Asian countries as well.

Suggestions on Strategy

To assist people in need costs money, and the amount can be astronomical if the goal is to built sustainable infrastructure and trained personnel for schools, clinics and orphanages, so that burgeoning nations may "take off" and show promise of sustained economic growth and profit for the investors. However, to attract investors to pay for projects suited to early stages of economic development is difficult. Investors usually follow other investors and may resist getting involved if they do not think that others will join them any time soon.[51]

Epidemic diseases like AIDS impact on all political, economic and cultural fronts, in terms of resource availability, resource allocation, and human rights. Africa needs foreign investment and responsible investors. But Africa also needs African leaders who are accountable, committed, and can manage their own affairs. These leaders must demonstrate willingness to lessen or eliminate disruptive intertribal wars and political instability that are costly and a deterrent to foreign investment. African leaders must also show they can protect revenues derived from their nations' natural resources, such as gold, diamonds, and oil, and invest them in their own country for the benefit of their citizens. Inappropriate or fraudulent use of natural resources can be an insurmountable obstacle to those otherwise willing to invest in Africa. On the other hand, there will never be enough money to build and maintain infrastructures, provide sanitation, clean water, education, and administer life-saving treatments to all who need it. But we can and should try to reach as many people as possible. It is our obligation as foreign investors – individuals, NGOs or government leaders – to clearly state what we can do, who we will target first, and to recognize what is beyond our will, ability, and resources. We should also be cautious about flashy programs, which are likely to fail or be meaningless, like the universal HIV testing announced in Lesotho that is not (at least yet) accompanied by strong antidiscrimination laws and universal access to effective treatment.[52]

Interventions to bring about change in countries with fundamentally different levels of economic structure and maturity may also encounter serious obstacles that are not recognized. For example, developed countries may favor introducing their own standards for education, social and cultural norms, bending as much as possible local rules, culture and traditions, believing as it may, that this will bring greater and better social and economic benefits. Alternatively, they may introduce standards that are different from those they commonly use to facilitate their partnerships with developing nations. In the former case, they may stand accused of neo-colonialism, and in the latter case their claims for equal and just partnerships with developing countries may be denounced as sheer propaganda and a cover for exploitation, particularly if the interventions fail to produce notable benefits. I believe it is critical to resolve these differences *at the start*, when the goal is to build suitable and sustainable progressive partnership with our African partners.

The key to a successful response to the AIDS epidemic in Africa is to construct achievable and realistic (probably limited) projects with measurable and transparent benchmarks, and to move from one benchmark to the other, focusing on each of them like a laser beam until all achieve their goals. Demonstration projects can be region-specific, problem-oriented, or both. As important, all partners involved in these projects must be able to find some personal benefits in them. Examples include sustainable mosquito treatment in specific regions to reduce the incidence of malaria, distribution of mosquito nets, water treatment, and drug affordability. Economist and advisor to Kofi Annan, Jeffrey Sachs, best illustrates what I have in mind in his plan, currently underway in the village of Sauri, Kenya, where AIDS has stricken 30% of the population, and the survivors did not have enough money for fertilizer or mosquito nets.[53] The villagers did not have cars or trucks, and half of these individuals had never made a phone call in their lives. With some modest resources, Sachs developed a plan to provide many of the things people in Sauri desperately need, i.e., a power line to a nearby town, a health clinic with a doctor and nurse, fertilizer, water storage facilities, mosquito nets, a cell phone, and a truck. The projected cost of this plan is $350,000 per year, or about $70 a person. The five-year plan has been funded, and is currently in its first year under the sponsorship of Columbia University's Earth Institute.[54] If it is successful and sustainable, the next step will be to replicate and scale it up. One of the major difficulties in such programs, however, is to ensure their financing at least until they are able to produce revenue on their own and continue to operate without outside resources. This last condition is critical for many reasons, but most importantly because Africa needs successful demonstration projects Africans can be proud of. They need projects that show the world and prove to themselves that they can and do improve the lives of their citizens.

The future of Africa ultimately rests in the hands of Africans. Given the poor implementation of the past grand projects financed by the World Bank and the International Monetary Fund, there is an urgent need for sustainable and suitable projects that can be used as models, to replace inefficient projects and "sloganing." Dr. Paul Farmer and collaborators at Partners In Health (PIH) has demonstrated that first world antiviral medication can be successfully delivered to people in the world's poorest countries. In rural Haiti, Farmer has shown that with a dedicated team of community health workers, nurses, doctors, laboratory technicians, social workers, and others, an integrated HIV prevention and treatment program can be successful. PIH has shown that it is possible to get first world results in HIV/AIDS prevention and treatment in a third world setting, and bring at least some of the benefits of modern science and medicine to those most in need. Instead of plundering poor nations, and use them as dumping grounds, Farmer insists, we must use the resources of rich nations to keep upping the living standards and health in poor nations by bringing life-saving treatment and hope. And most importantly, he actually does it.[55]

Of course, sub-Saharan Africa is not Haiti, and no one solution fits all. For the 48 countries, 800 languages, and more than 1000 ethnic groups in Africa, many projects are needed to address specific health problems and conditions. A requisite, however, is that African nations make every reasonable effort to promote and defend human rights. All African nations have signed the Universal Declaration of Human Rights, and it is unacceptable that governments can still stand by and watch while people's rights are violated, like in Malawi where women are used as "trading tools" by their fathers, who unapologetically say they own their daughters and can sell them (at the young age of 11 or 12 years old) to old men, in order to pay for their debts. As Jonathan Mann stated, health and human rights are "inextricably linked,"[56] and only when they are taken together is human well being likely to be advanced. As I have already emphasized, the health and human rights dyad has real meaning worldwide. Hiding behind culture and tradition to avoid addressing inequality and discrimination is simply not acceptable as a matter of human rights and dignity. As the editor of the *Lancet* put it in the context of WHO's mission:

> The progressive realization of human rights must be a pillar of WHO's work. Currently the agency has shied away from a strong rights-based approach to health. It is deemed too political, too invasive of member-states' sovereignty. Yet if the Millennium Declaration Goals are the spine of WHO's work, human rights must be its moral skin. WHO must be an activist for the intrinsic dignity and well-being of individuals worldwide. Without that coherent moral vision, the agency's public-health work will be little more than abstract series of statistics.[57]

Finally, good governance is necessary for success in stemming the AIDS epidemic. But so long as African nations remain emotionally and psychologically indebted to other countries, particularly former colonizers, they will resist programs that can make a significant difference in the lives of their citizens. South African president Thabo Mbeki, for example, may continue to insist that poverty, not AIDS, is the cause of most health problems in South Africa, but he may not continue to overlook that AIDS kills those who are HIV infected, and view as a Western (American) ploy the scientific explanation that HIV causes AIDS.[58] When African nations accept within their own national conscience that they stand equal with any other countries, they may more likely form vital partnerships with foreign countries, and engage in new strategies, ideas, and programs to help arrest the AIDS epidemic.

Obviously, nation states cannot (and should not) be manipulated and coerced (by military or other interventions) to adopt preventive and curative health measures regardless of benefit, and the commerce model or the belief that the common interest is best served by allowing individual participants and nations to pursue their self-interests cannot be defended in good faith. The charitable or humanitarian model offers solutions to treatment access and prevention that have been unacceptable to South Africa and would probably be also unacceptable to most African nations. Nonetheless, we do not have to contemplate the humanitarian model to observe that rich countries have obligations too. As philosopher and scholar, Kwame Anthony Appiah, has observed, "we are not in danger of being excessively generous. ...If there are people without basic entitlements – and there are billions of them – we know that, collectively, we are not meeting our obligations." His conclusion is echoed in my essay and concludes it:

> Africa has been left behind, and it is Africa that presents the greatest

challenge to our development experts – and to our sense of our global obligations. Faced with impossible demands, we are likely to throw up our hands in horror. But the obligations we have are not monstrous or unreasonable. They do not require us to abandon our own lives. What's wanted ... is the exercise of reason, not just explosions of feeling.[59]

Notes

[1]Sub-Saharan Africa is comprised of 48 nations, 42 in the mainland, 4 island nations in the southwest Indian Ocean and two island nations in the Atlantic Ocean. In this essay I focus on the 42 nations which are south of the Sahara Desert, on the mainland.

[2]Lawrence K. Altman and Elisabeth Rosenthal, "U.N. Strengthens Call for a Global Battle Against AIDS," *New York Times*, June 3, 2006.

[3]Nicholas D. Kristof, "A Mother of Two," *New York Times*, May 28, 2006.

[4]Jeffrey D. Sachs, *The End of Poverty: Economic Possibilities for our Time* (New York: The Penguin Press, 2005).

[5]Stephen Lewis, *Race Against Time* (Toronto: House of Anansi Press Inc., 2005), 148.

[6]International Treatment Preparedness Coalition, ITPC, "Missing the Target: A Report on HIV/AIDS Treatment Access from the Frontlines, November 28, 2005," http: //www.aidstreatmentaccess.org.

[7]"Maintaining Anti-AIDS Commitment Post '3 by 5,'" *The Lancet* 366 (2005): 1828. I would like to acknowledge Dr. Lee Jonk Wook's contribution to this program. Dr. Wook who died on May 22, 2006, enthusiastically championed the "3 by 5" AIDS treatment program. Writing the obituary, Laurence K. Altman of the *New York Times* stated (citing Dr. Foege), "the failure to achieve the '3 by 5' goal was insignificant compared to the courage of promoting a vision of what the world should be doing." (*New York Times*, May 23, 2006). Obviously we should credit Dr. Wook for his vision and support, and we may wonder who at WHO will be able and willing to play such a strong advocacy role. But vision, although important, is not enough. We also need to fulfill our obligations and comparable resources.

[8]Global Aids Alliance, http://www.globalaidalliance.org.

[9]Leonard Rubenstein, Executive Director of Physicians for Human Rights (oral communication, 4th Annual Conference on HIV/AIDS in Africa: Taking Action, University of Pennsylvania, January 25, 2002.

[10]Shreekanth Chaguturu and Snigdha Vallabhabemi, "Aiding and Abetting – Nurses Crisis at Home and Abroad," *New England Journal of Medicine* 353 (2005): 1761-63. See also Fizhugh Mullan, "The Metrics of the Physician Brain-Drain," *New England Journal of Medicine* 353 (2005): 1810-18; and Lincoln C. Chen and Jo Ivey Boufford, "Fatal Blows – Doctors on the Move," *New Englan Journal of Medicine* 353 (2005): 1850-52.

[11]Sharon LaFraniere, "U.N. Envoy Sharply Criticizes South Africa AIDS Program," *New York Times*, October 25, 2005. See also John B. Jemmott III, "A Setback in AIDS Fight," *Philadelphia Inquirer*, May 10, 2006.

[12] Celia. W. Dugger, "Devastated by AIDS, Africa Sees Life Expectancy Plunge," *New York Times*, July 16, 2005; M. Wines, "Women in Lesotho Become Easy Prey for HIV," *New York Times*, July 20, 2004.

[13] Mandela's speech is available at http://www.aidstrust.org.

[14] Available at http://www.cnn.com/ALLPOLITICS/inauguration/2001/trascripts/template.html.

[15] Available at http://www.clintonfoundation.org/legacy/021700-speech-by-president-at-opening-of-africaSummit.htm.

[16] Elie Wiesel, Foreword to *The Nazi Doctors and the Nuremberg Code*, ed. George J. Annas and Michael A. Grodin (New York: Oxford University Press, 1992), vii-ix.

[17] Jonathan Glover, *Humanity: A Moral History of the Twentieth Century* (Yale University Press, 1999).

[18] Supra, note 13. Cameron publicly disclosed his HIV status to help "destigmatize" the disease.

[19] Supra, note 14.

[20] Anthony Lewis, "Africa on the Agenda," *New York Times,* May 19, 2001.

[21] Barton Gellman, "AIDS is declared Threat to Security," *Washington Post*, April 30, 2000.

[22] UN Security Council Session on AIDS in Africa, *Fighting AIDS Together* (Washington, D.C.: Office of the Vice-President, 2000).

[23] Jennifer Logan Coyle, "The Arc of Justice: The Ethical Implications of Framing the HIV/AIDS Pandemic as a National Security Threat: An Annotated Bibliography," *International Quarterly of Community Health Education* 23 (2004/2005):39-61.

[24] President George W. Bush's address to the United Nations General Assembly, June 2001, available at http://www.whitehouse.gov/news/releases/2001/11/20011110-3.html.

[25] "President Commemorates 60th Anniversary of V-J Day," http://www.whitehouse.gov/new/releases/2005/08. See also "President Commemorates Veterans Day, Discusses War on Terror," http://www.whitehouse.gov/new/releases/2005.

[26] Don Noah and George Fidas, *The Global Infectious Disease Threat and its Implications for the United States* (Washington, DC: CIA, Office of Public Affairs, 2000).

[27] In an article on the Hobbesian model, "The Realist Persuasion," *Sunday Boston Globe*, November 6, 2005, Andrew J. Bacevich explains that "realist is the idea that America should be guided by strategic self-interest and that moral considerations are secondary at best." In another article on the same model, "What Turned Brent Scowcroft Against the Bush Administration?" Jeffrey Goldberg makes a similar argument (*The New Yorker*, October 31, 2005).

[28] Médecins Sans Frontières, "Mission Statement," http://www.msf.org.

[29] Tina Rosenberg, *New York Times Magazine*, January 28, 2001.

[30] "Accelerating Access Initiative: Widening Access to Care and Support for People Living with HIV/AIDS," Progress Report, June 2002, available online through the WHO website. It is to be noted that Pfizer was already engaged in controversy in South Africa when the drug company wanted to donate its powerful and expensive antifungal, Diflucan, for treatment of cryptococcal meningitis, a deadly AIDS related infection. Yet, donation was not acceptable to the South African government because of fear that it might not be sustained. It also created a dangerous dependency to the branded drug. See also Kevin

Outterson, "Pharmaceutical Arbitrage: Balancing Access and Innovation in International Prescription Drug Markets," *Yale Journal of Health Policy, Law and Ethics*, 5 (2005): 193-291.

[31] "Secure the Future. Care and Support for Women and Children in Africa with HIV/AIDS: Creating a Legacy of Hope in Sub-Saharan Africa, Bristol-Myers Squibb," http://www.securethefuture.com. Today, BMS and its partners, including Baylor College of Medicine, Baylor International Pediatric AIDS Initiative, Catholic Medical Mission Board, Harvard AIDS institute, UNAIDS, the Center for Interdisciplinary Research on AIDS, and others have a number of programs in place or in process of being developed with different goals. These programs explore research, prevention and treatment to combat the disease and its effects. BMS and partners work with local governments of countries like Botswana, Lesotho, Namibia, South Africa and Swaziland. See http://www.securethefuture.com.

[32] Supra, note 2.

[33] Available at http://www.msf.org.au.

[34] Renee Fox, "Medical Humanitarianism and Human Rights: Reflections on Doctors Without Borders and Doctors of the World," in *Health and Human Rights: A Reader*, ed. Jonathan M. Mann, Sofia Gruskin (New York: Routledge Press, 1999), pp.417-438.

[35] Jonathan M. Mann, Lawrence Gostin, Sofia Gruskin et al., "Health and Human Rights," in Mann and Gruskin, eds., *Health and Human Rights*, 7-20.

[36] Nelson Mandela, "Closing Remarks" (XIV International AIDS Conference, Barcelona, Spain, July 15, 2002), http://ww.aidstrust.org.

[37] Sharon LaFraniere, "Forced to Marry Before Puberty. African Girls Pay Lasting Price," *Sunday New York Times*, November 27, 2005.

[38] Seth Mydans, "Shunned, Women with HIV Join Forces in Vietnam," *New York Times*, May 28, 2006.

[39] Paul Farmer, *Infections and Inequalities: The Modern Plagues* (Berkeley: University of California Press, 2001). Paul Farmer, *Pathologies of Power: Health, Human Rights and the New War on the Poor* (Berkeley: University of California Press, 2003).

[40] Evelyne Shuster, "The UN's Plea on Guantanamo," *New York Times*, February 20, 2006.

[41] Supra, note 2.

[42] Laurence K. Altman, "AIDS Goal Missed, but Effort by UN Branch is Praised," *New York Times*, November 29, 2005.

[43] Jim Yong Kim and Charlie Gilks, "Scaling up Treatment – Why We Can't Wait," *New England Journal of Medicine* 353 (2005): 2392-94.

[44] "Pression en Algerie: Loi du 23 Fevrier 2005," *Le Nouvel Observateur*, November 30, 2005.

[45] Raymond Aron, *The Dawn of Universal History* (New York: Basic Books Press, 2002).

[46] Edward M. Connor, Rhoda S. Sperling, Richard Gelber, et al., "Reduction of Maternal-Infant Transmission of Human Immuno-Deficiency Virus Type 1 with Zidovudine Treatment," *New England Journal of Medicine* 331 (1994): 1173-1180.

[47] Peter Lurie and Sydney M. Wolff, "Unethical Trials of Interventions To Reduce Perinatal Transmission of the Human Immunodeficiency Virus in Developing Countries," *New England Journal of Medicine* 337 (1997): 853-856.

[48] Marcia Angell, "The Ethics of Clinical Research in The Third World," *New England Journal of Medicine* 337 (1997): 847-49.

[49] Leonard H. Glantz, George J. Annas, et al., "Research in Developing Countries: Taking 'Benefit' Seriously," *The Hasting Center Report*, 28 (1998): 38-42.

[50] Harold Varmus and David Satcher, "Ethical Complexities of Conducting Research in Developing Countries," *New England Journal of Medicine* 337 (1997): 1003-1005. Antony S. Fauci, "The AIDS Epidemic," *New England Journal of Medicine* 341 (1999): 1046-1050.

[51] Jon Cohen, "The New World of Global Health," *Science* 311 (2006): 162-167.

[52] John Donnelly, "Dire Situation, Drastic Measures: AIDS Testing Urged for All in Ravaged Nation," *Sunday Boston Globe*, October 23, 2005.

[53] John Cassidy, "Always With Us: Jeffrey Sachs's Plan to Eradicate World Poverty," *New Yorker*, November 11, 2005. Available at **www.newyorker.com/printables/critics/ o50411crbo_books**. See also Sachs, *The End of Poverty*.

[54] Sachs, *The End of Poverty*.

[55] Paul Farmer, et al., "Community-Based Approaches to HIV Treatment in Resource-Poor Settings," *Lancet* 358 (2001): 404-09. Patrice Severe, Paul Leger, Macarthur Charles, et al., "Antiretroviral Therapy in a Thousand Patients with AIDS in Haiti," *New England Journal of Medicine* 353 (2005): 2325-34.

[56] Supra, note 34.

[57] Richard Horton, "WHO: Strengthening the Road to Renewal," *The Lancet* 367 (2006): 1793-95.

[58] As the editor of *The Lancet*, Richard Horton, put it: "One of the major stumbling blocks [to effectively deal with the AIDS epidemic] remains the lack of a strong leadership that delivers clear messages. Government officials need to overcome their complacency, their scientific opinions and reactions to the HIV/AIDS epidemic," *The Lancet*, 367 (2006): 1629.

[59] Kwame Anthony Appiah, *Cosmopolitanism. Ethics in a World of Strangers* (New York: W.W. Norton Co., 2006), 170, 172, 173.

CHAPTER 6

Stigma and the Political Economy of Disease: The Neglected Dimension of Interventions to Reduce HIV/AIDS Stigma

LAURA MCGOUGH

I want to start with two quotations from contemporary Mali, in which two informants explained the origin and transmission of AIDS via young Malians who migrate to Côte d'Ivoire and contract HIV/AIDS there:

> This is what I have heard. I myself was in Côte d'Ivoire and even saw a child who was with a white person and who slept with a dog. They say that she became infected by the dog. If these girls come and sleep with our young men, that's how they get AIDS. That is the information I have. (Village A, father of out-of-school girl, 54 years old [FGD])

> AIDS? Aagh! [laughs] it is the illness of dogs. Because white people get their dogs ready and then suggest to girls who are looking for money – large sums of money – that they have sex with their dogs and so this is how they get AIDS. It is not an illness sent from God but from men and it is white people that have brought it to us. In this way they [the girls] come back, ever so charming, and they will seduce men easily – who in turn will be infected if they sleep together. (Village B, head of the hunters (gatekeeper), 90-years-old [IDI]).[1]

These descriptions of possible mechanisms of transmission elucidate a range of anxieties and perceived vulnerabilities: the economic vulnerability of young Malian females, forced to trade sex for money; the vulnerability of the Malian economy, whose workers must migrate to neighboring Côte d'Ivoire to support themselves and families back home; the anxieties about corrupt and morally decadent whites, who still exercise political and economic influence in the post-colonial era. Fear of biological contagion incorporates fears about other kinds of contagion: moral, cultural, political, and social.[2] The anthropologist who collected this data, Sarah Castle, underscored the importance of addressing the social context of infection, in addition to factual misperceptions about HIV transmission and acquisition, in order to develop interventions to reduce HIV/AIDS stigma. "In particular," she argues, "the community needs to openly confront fears about labour migration and the re-integration of returned migrants so that they can be accommodated sensitively within village life rather than reacted to with blame and mistrust."[3]

I have chosen to start with this ethnographic account of AIDS stigma in rural Mali because it nicely illustrates how social scientists have recently defined the problem of stigma: stigma is linked to broader patterns of social inequality, to political and economic power, and to domination. Accounts of disease origins and transmission are often situated within a larger political, economic, or military framework: disease carries this larger symbolic weight as a representation of national vulnerability.[4] As public health officials have highlighted the importance of reducing stigma to combat the AIDS epidemic, researchers have been re-investigating the nature of stigma, producing major new revisions and reinterpretations of Erving Goffman's classic 1963 work.[5] New work has highlighted the strengths and limitations of Goffman's approach, in particular noting how he focused on the individual, rather than larger social groups. For Link and Phelan, for example, the crucial research question is to investigate "how culturally created categories arise and how they are sustained."[6] Furthermore, stigma is embedded in broader patterns of power and domination: to understand how stigma is created and reproduced, it is necessary to study social inequality in a given society.[7] Despite the new theoretical work on stigma, however, few interventions for STDs or HIV/AIDS have made use of these theoretical insights. Most of the interventions to reduce HIV/AIDS stigma have focused on information alone, that is, on increasing knowledge and correcting misperceptions about the ways in which HIV is transmitted and acquired.[8] Despite more than a decade of research about the "KAP/gap" (the gap among knowledge, attitudes and practice), stigma interventions have continued to focus on knowledge alone.[9]

AIDS stigma has been identified as one of the principal obstacles to HIV testing worldwide, as well as an obstacle to seeking treatment until patients have reached an advanced stage of disease, often with CD4 cell counts at

50 or below.[10] There is, however, some reason for optimism. As antiretro-viral therapy becomes increasingly available through major international programs (such as the Global Fund, the World Bank, and the President's Emergency Plan for AIDS Relief, or PEPFAR), as the disease is no longer a death sentence and patients are restored to a healthy appearance and pro-ductive life, AIDS stigma is expected to decrease. As Arachu Castro and Paul Farmer have recently argued, the major impediment to testing thus far has been the lack of treatment, not stigma.[11] With increased access to treatment, it is reasonable to anticipate that stigma will decline, at least partially. But the stigma associated with AIDS has never been a product only of the disease's fatal consequences. In the United States, for example, HIV/AIDS stigma persists despite the widespread availability of treatment (although access for the poor is limited, a point I will come back to later).[12] The association of the disease with sexual transmission, including homo-sexual transmission, and with injection drug use, explains the persistence of stigma. Furthermore, the concentration of HIV/AIDS among African-Americans no doubt contributes to the stigma, as well as to the perception by some that HIV was produced in government laboratories as a form of genocide against blacks.[13] The recent debate about "conspiracy theories" of HIV/AIDS among African-Americans[14] is simply the latest episode in a continuing history of stigma associated with sexually transmitted diseases, even after the availability of medical therapies.

The goal of this paper is two-fold: (1) to examine historical precedents of how stigma associated with sexually transmitted diseases has been re-produced, despite changes in medical therapy; and (2) to encourage public health professionals to use this information for the delivery of AIDS treat-ment programs. I focus on two historical examples: the discovery of a variety of "cures" for syphilis, more commonly called the French disease or the pox, in 16th century Europe; and the development of penicillin for the treatment of syphilis and gonorrhea during World War II. Neither of these examples is perfectly analogous to the situation of HIV/AIDS in sub-Saharan Africa. For one thing, syphilis was acknowledged as a po-tentially fatal disease during both the 16th and 20th centuries, but not considered to be a "death sentence" for all who contracted it, as is the case with untreated HIV/AIDS. Treatment for the pox during the 16th cen-tury consisted of mercury, guaiacum, and a variety of ointments and herbal treatments which would not, by present-day standards, be considered clinically efficacious. Nonetheless, contemporaries regarded them as efficacious, and syphilis was widely regarded as a "cured" disease by the mid-sixteenth century. As the following historical examples will show, when treatment becomes available, stigma can shift from the entire group of patients to certain sub-groups, those who do not respond medically to treatment – the poor and marginalized, females, and the "guilty" who sell sex or are perceived as leading immoral lives. The "diseased" remain powerful symbols of a nation's vulnerability long after treatment is available.

Stigma and the French Disease in early modern Italy

Historical research shows how stigma associated with a disease can change over time, with different groups of people and cultural attributes becoming the focus of anxiety. During the first European syphilis epidemic of the late fifteenth century,[15] Europeans struggled to understand this disease, including whether it was a new disease. By borrowing the imagery of leprosy, writers, painters, and physicians simultaneously made syphilis more familiar and hence less threatening to their contemporaries. Even if leprosy was considered repugnant, it had also become less common during this period. Another means of coping with syphilis was to displace blame for the disease on "Others," notably foreigners (hence the Italians called it the French disease, the French the Neapolitan disease, etc.), American Indians, and Jews.[16] By the mid-sixteenth century, however, attention shifted towards prostitutes and "loose women" who were encouraged to repent and enter convents dedicated to Mary Magdalene. Several sixteenth-century convents for "fallen women" began with former syphilis patients from *ospedali degli incurabili* (hospitals of the incurables, primarily but not exclusively for syphilis patients)[17]

A thriving medical marketplace in syphilis cures during the late sixteenth and seventeenth centuries convinced the early modern European public that the disease was curable.[18] Whether or not these therapies are judged efficacious by today's standards, they were regarded as such by their contemporaries. Physicians or licensed healers who sold remedies to cure syphilis were bound by contracts: if the patient did not recover, he or she could sue and demand compensation for monies spent.[19] Despite the availability of some kind of medical therapy for virtually every income level, the stigma and shame associated with syphilis persisted.[20] Fear of death and disfigurement, which had diminished as medical therapies became available, were not the only reasons for the stigma of syphilis. Equally important were the quality of care and privacy offered to the patient, which varied with income level. The wealthy could afford private physicians and confidential treatment, while the poor had to make their disease publicly known in order to access public charity.[21] Furthermore, the more difficult the disease was to treat, the more exotic (and expensive) the therapeutic ingredients became. Instead of just simple chicken fat, one writer recommended the fat of a badger, bear, and goose, along with the blood of a male pig, to cure the French disease.[22] Only persons of "quality" would have been able to afford these expensive ingredients.

The stigma associated with syphilis persisted because it was embedded in wider patterns of domination, subordination, and social inequality, as theorists such as Richard Parker and Peter Aggleton have argued. Part of the problem was that the disease came to be associated with sexual activity, but that association was more problematic for women than for men, for the poor than for the rich. In early modern England, for example, the Lock Asylum released men after their treatment with mercury, but required that women remain in the institution after treatment for a period of moral reform: a two-stage process for women, a one-stage process for men.[23] In Venice, the Hospital of the *Incurabili* used the same procedure: medical treatment for men, medical and moral treatment for women.[24] Transmission of syphilis was blamed on women,[25] who were already devalued as women, and then associated with disease.

Although the evidence suggests that syphilis was a widespread disease in early modern Venice, not confined to sub-groups such as prostitutes and soldiers, the public and the medical profession increasingly linked prostitution with the disease. Witchcraft trials provide some evidence of how this process of linking prostitution (or immoral behavior) to medical diagnoses of syphilis worked. For example, Bellina Loredana stood trial on charges of having used witchcraft to make another woman, a prostitute named Angela Castellana, get sick with syphilis and die.[26] In defense of the accused, a physician called in as an expert witness testified that she could not be held responsible for Castellana's death. Like most other physicians of his time, this university-educated doctor firmly believed in the possibility that witchcraft could cause disease, and could even cause a disease such as syphilis.[27] However, if the person who contracted syphilis was a prostitute, demonic causation was unnecessary; prostitutes always died of syphilis. As a physician explained, Angela Castellana

> for her entire life was a public prostitute making her body available to everyone; and because of this she was already for many years full of the French disease sores (*gomme*) and other incurable diseases; where [at the hospital of San Giovanni and Paolo] she died miserably because of these aforesaid illnesses not for another [reason], as is usual for similar prostitutes and this is well-known, and obvious and thus the truth.[28]

Incurable cases of syphilis did not cause physicians to rethink the system of medications and therapies they offered to patients. Instead, incurable cases were blamed on patients' immoral behavior. Even a nobleman's life was subject to scrutiny for immoral behavior if he was unresponsive to medical treatment. The nobleman Andrea Marcello, who had abandoned his long-term girlfriend Camilla Savioni after 10 or 11 years, was treated several times for syphilis, but his condition progressed. His family feared that his abandoned lover had practiced witchcraft to make him sick and die, out of revenge and a desire to inherit his house, which, they alleged, she had made him bequeath to her in his will. Physicians' testimony was divided between those who would and those who would not rule out witchcraft, but in the end the physicians who argued that witchcraft did not play a role in this case persuaded the court to acquit Camilla Savioni. The decisive testimony implicated the nobleman's immoral behavior, rather than witchcraft, as the main cause of disease:

> it appears that the infirmity of this Signor Andrea Marcello was believed to be a disease that the doctors call epilepsy, great in itself, but seeing that this gentleman was also infected with *morbo gallico*, and seeing that he led a most irregular life, as regards to witchcraft we do not see the effects that for this illness we could suspect witchcraft. And we conclude that it was the natural illnesses of *morbo gallico* and *mal caduco*.[29]

Andrea's "most irregular life" figured prominently in his diagnosis. Despite living in an era when syphilis, according to contemporaries, had been "cured," stigma did not abate, but intensified for certain sub-groups. Therapeutic failures were blamed on patients' moral failings.

Syphilis, or French disease, also bore enormous symbolic weight since its very name referred to the military and political vulnerability of the

Italian peninsula. Despite differences in medical and popular opinion about where the disease ultimately originated, whether it was entirely new or a recurrent older disease, whether it was cannibalism, a conjunction of the planets, or sexual intercourse between a prostitute and soldiers which sparked an epidemic, all agreed that the recent outbreak coincided with the French invasion of Italy and the subsequent humiliations of the Italian Wars (1494-1530). This focus on the French invasion did not abate with time, as the Italian peninsula never regained its autonomy and strength. On the contrary, by the mid-sixteenth century the French invasion came to be seen as turning-point in the political and military history of the Italian city-states, as Florence and Milan fell to Habsburg power. The French disease was a visible sign of political and military vulnerability, a continuing weakness in the face of ever-greater Turkish strength. The stigma associated with the French disease continued during this period, not just because it was associated with the sexuality or immoral behavior of individuals, but because of the potential impact of that behavior on the political strength of the society as a whole. Syphilis literally embodied Italian vulnerability.

Outside of Italy, syphilis or the "pox" carried an equally rich set of meanings. From Shakespeare's *Timon of Athens* to Rabelais's *Pantagruel*, the pox appeared frequently in literature, far more often than any disease except the plague.[30] As Susan Sontag famously noticed, illness serves as a powerful metaphor during any age. The metaphoric associations of a given illness make the experience of that illness more difficult, she argued: "My point is that illness is not a metaphor, and that the most truthful way of regarding illness – and the healthiest way of being ill – is one most purified of, most resistant to, metaphoric thinking."[31] From the point of view of the person who experiences illness, Sontag's analysis yields many useful insights. But given the ubiquity with which illness (especially but not only sexually transmitted diseases) becomes stigmatized and embedded in larger discourses about gender, social relations, power, and even political and military strength,[32] it might be useful to pause for a moment and ask whether the most useful strategy in combating stigma is to combat these metaphors. Most public health interventions have followed Sontag's approach and tried to replace cultural associations of disease with correct medical knowledge. But as I have already argued, this approach operates on the assumption that stigma is simply incorrect knowledge, an idea challenged by recent works.[33]

The example of syphilis in early modern Europe provides a few historical lessons about the persistence of stigma when treatment is available for STDs. First, treatment of the same quality is seldom available equally to all patients; the availability of "high-quality care," with greater guarantees of confidentiality, enables stigma to persist among the less affluent and more socially marginalized groups. Second, in order to explain treatment failure, physicians and the general public blame the patients' behavior. Third and finally, the disease itself is a powerful symbol (in the Italian context, it represented political and military vulnerability).

Throughout sub-Saharan Africa, HIV/AIDS has generated a rich set of meanings. In parts of Ethiopia, for example, AIDS is seen as a punishment from God because people have distanced themselves too much from religion.[34] The idea that the disease is a punishment for having broken a moral code is common throughout Africa and other parts of the world.[35] Gender and class play an important role in stigma and assigning blame for the transmission of HIV, with women (especially young women) being held responsible in addition to wealthy men, who can afford to take several lovers. Women's poverty sometimes excuses them from blame, although some women continue to be regarded as promiscuous and blameworthy.[36] AIDS as a "foreign" disease plays a double role in Africa: Africans often associate the disease with white people and homosexuals, including recurrent rumors about the disease having been intentionally introduced by the CIA or other Western agency,[37] while at the same time many Africans are aware that they are associated with and blamed for the disease in the Western media, thereby becoming entangled with broader issues of economic globalization, development and the role of donors, and political power.[38] The broader meanings attached to disease, especially but not only sexually transmitted diseases, make it difficult to eliminate stigma, even when public health officials consciously try to reduce the impact of stigma, as the following example will show.

Penicillin during World War II

The experiences of wartime VD control have been explored at length by Allan Brandt and others, so the following description is a brief synopsis.[39] After an initial media campaign to control prostitution, especially near military bases, and the development of Rapid Treatment Centers for civilians, public health officials realized that their campaigns had erroneously associated all venereal diseases with prostitution. The result was that the general public was reluctant to go to the Rapid Treatment Centers. Their own public health campaign had contributed to the stigmatization of disease and inadvertently discouraged the majority of sexual contacts (who were not prostitutes) from seeking treatment. The blunder led to a new campaign that emphasized how anyone, even a woman who "looks clean," could spread venereal disease, that referred to the Rapid Treatment Centers in urban areas as "hospitals," and created a "hospital atmosphere" in them.[40]

In practice, military and public health policy primarily focused on females as vectors of disease. The campaign to eliminate prostitution near military bases disproportionately targeted working-class women and women of color. One woman was arrested and detained for suspicious behavior because she was eating lunch alone at a public lunch-counter.[41] VD posters and the public health campaign operated within a wider social, cultural, and political environment in which male sexuality was celebrated, while women were encouraged to be in supportive, secondary roles.[42] Furthermore, the campaign to control VD operated in a larger political framework in which foreign women, the enemy, were represented as dangerous not only in their ability to spread disease, but also to spread rumors that would undermine the war effort. Images of the seductive female represented multiple threats to the individual and national health. Men apparently internalized this message. At a Conference of Preventive Medicine at Johns Hopkins University in February 1945, Capt. Larimore explained why so many men became infected when they returned home: "They say that when they are overseas their medical officers and commanding officers all told them, 'When you were back in the States the girls were clean, and you could take a chance but, soldier, while you are over here don't take any chances. If you do you will get burned because these girls over here are all infected.' The result is that they come back home with the feeling that the girls back here are clean and they don't need to worry about exposing themselves with impunity, and without regard to prophylaxis."[43] As mentioned earlier, it is difficult to remove sexually transmitted diseases from the larger social, political, and economic issues in which sexual relationships, and hence the transmission of STDs, are situated.

Stigma Interventions in Public Health

So what do we do with information about the perpetuation of stigma when treatment becomes available? Throw our hands up in despair? On the contrary, it is worth using the historical knowledge, that stigma does not disappear when treatment becomes available (especially when it becomes available only to some),[44] to decide which strategies are most effective in mitigating the impact of stigma.

Let's return to the example of Mali with which I started. Recall the stories about how HIV/AIDS was transmitted through sexual unions between white people's dogs and female migrants working temporarily in Côte d'Ivoire. Let's take Paul Farmer's notion of social vulnerability – which I would extend to include political and economic vulnerability – and read this ethnography through this lens. Paul Farmer has argued persuasively that the term "risk groups" inappropriately locates control within individuals and ignores the inequalities of power that make some groups more vulnerable than others.[45] Farmer's concept of "social vulnerability" to HIV/AIDS, which highlights structural inequalities, is a useful idea to bring to the development of stigma interventions. What I want to do is take his idea one step farther: not only do public health professionals and social scientists need to look at social vulnerabilities rather than risk groups, but also we (that is, social scientists and public health workers) need to use ethnographic information about HIV/AIDS as an insight into local people's perceptions of their own social, economic and political vulnerability, rather than as a catalog of misperceptions about HIV transmission.

Like people from many different cultures and historical contexts, Malians project their anxieties about their vulnerabilities as a people into their narratives of disease. The labor migration of young females, the political and economic hegemony of European and American power, the power differences between wealthy white or Ivorian men versus young, impoverished Malian women – all these political, economic, and social vulnerabilities make Malians as a group more vulnerable to HIV/AIDS. Instead of regarding disease origin and transmission stories as products of exotic local culture, it is more useful to view them as responses to perceived and often actual power inequalities and vulnerabilities that Malians experience and recognize as real threats to the public health of their communities. Rather than focusing on wiping out stigma per se, it might be more useful to employ ethnographic analysis to learn more about which groups are perceived as vulnerable and require more support. Instead of public health interventions to reduce stigma, it might be useful to think about how to develop public health conversations with local communities about political, social, and economic vulnerability to HIV/AIDS, and ways to reduce it.[46] It is especially important to place ethnography about Africa in a political and economic context, thus countering the long history (and current practice) of reducing complex problems in Africa to expressions of a "backward" culture, and ignoring the political and economic systems that reproduce inequality and stigma.[47]

Notes

[1]Sarah Castle, "Rural Children's Attitudes to People with HIV/AIDS in Mali: The Causes of Stigma," *Culture, Health & Sexuality* 6 (2004): 11.

[2]Mary Douglas, *Purity and Danger: An Analysis of Concepts of Pollution and Taboo* (New York and London: Routledge and Kegan Paul, 1966).

[3]Castle, "Rural Children's Attitudes to People with HIV/AIDS," 15.

[4]Paul Farmer, *AIDS and Accusation: Haiti and the Geography of Blame* (Berkeley: University of California Press, 1992); Leslie Ann Jeffrey, *Sex and Borders: Gender, National Identity, and Prostitution Policy in Thailand* (Chiang Mai, Thailand: Silkworm Books, 2002).

[5] Erving Goffman, *Stigma: Notes on the Management of a Spoiled Identity* (Englewood Cliffs, NJ: Prentice Hall, 1963).

[6]B. G. Link and J. C. Phelan, "Conceptualizing Stigma," *Annual Review of Sociology* 27 (2001): 363-85. On the cultural construction of "risk groups" and HIV/AIDS, see Carl Kendall, "The Construction of Risk in AIDS Control Programs," in *Conceiving Sexuality: Approaches to Sex Research in a Postmodern World*, ed. Richard G. Parker and John H. Gagnon (New York and London: Routledge, 1995).

[7]Richard Parker and Peter Aggleton, "HIV and AIDS-Related Stigma and Discrimination," *Social Science & Medicine* 57 (2003): 13-24.

[8]Lisanne Brown, Kate Macintyre, and Lea Trujillo, "Interventions to Reduce HIV/AIDS Stigma: What Have We Learned?" *AIDS Education and Prevention* 15: 1 (2003): 49-69. Not other peer-reviewed stigma interventions have been published since this article. I contacted Lisanne Brown via email to see if she is working on new stigma interventions and she is not. A search of the CRISP index revealed more than 50 studies-in-progress on stigma, mostly from the fields of psychology and social psychology. These studies did not involve the larger political, economic, and social context of stigma, or the metaphors of disease.

[9]The KAP/gap refers to the widely observed discrepancy between people's knowledge and attitudes about health versus their actual practices. The phrase was first used in reproductive health. See for example John Bangaarts, "The KAP-Gap and the Unmet Need for Contraception," *Population and Development Review* 17 (1991): 293-313;

Charles F. Westoff, "Is the KAP-Gap Real?" *Population and Development Review* 14 (1988): 225-232. The phrase KAP-gap has been used in the HIV/AIDS field to refer to a common problem in HIV prevention efforts in which increased information about prevention (such as condoms to prevent HIV transmission) does not necessarily result in behavior change. The literature on this topic is vast; see for example, C. Kendall, "The Construction of Risk in AIDS Control Programs: Theoretical Bases and Popular Responses," in *Conceiving Sexuality: Approaches to Sex in a Postmodern World*, ed. R. G. Parker and J. H. Gagnon (New York: Routledge, 1995), 249-258; B. G. Schoepf, "International AIDS Research in Anthropology: Taking a Critical Perspective on the Crisis," *Annual Review of Anthropology* 30 (2001): 335-361; James P. Stanbury and Manuel Sierra, "Risks, Sigma and Honduran Garifuna Conceptions of HIV/AIDS," *Social Science and Medicine* 59 (2004): 457-471, esp. 458.

[10] Ronald O. Valdiserri, "HIV/AIDS Stigma: An Impediment to Public Health," *American Journal of Public Health* 93 (2002): 341-2; "Stepping Back from the Edge: The Pursuit of Antiretroviral Therapy in Botswana, South Africa, and Uganda," *UNAIDS* April 2004.

[11] Arachu Castro and Paul Farmer, "Understanding and Addressing AIDS-Related Stigma: From Anthropological Theory to Clinical Practice in Haiti," *American Journal of Public Health* 95 (2005): 53-59.

[12] "National Survey Shows Fear of HIV/AIDS Stigma Persists," *AIDS Policy & Law* (2004): 2. Stigma has decreased in the U.S. during the 1990s, but certainly not disappeared. In 1999, for example, approximately 16.3% of Americans surveyed agreed with the statement that "the names of people with AIDS should be made public so that others can avoid them," compared with 28.8% of Americans surveyed in 1991. See Gregory M. Herek, John P. Capitanio, and Keith Wideman, "HIV-Related Stigma and Knowledge in the United States: Prevalence and Trends, 1991-1999," *American Journal of Public Health* 92 (2002): 371-377.

[13] Laura Bogart and Sheryl Thorburn, "Are HIV/AIDS Conspiracy Beliefs a Barrier to HIV Prevention Among African Americans?" *Journal of Acquired Immune Deficiency Syndrome* 38 (2005): 213-218.

[14] For commentary on the study by Bogart and Thorburn, see "Clearing the Myths of Time: Tuskegee Revisited," *The Lancet Infectious Diseases* 5 (2005): 127.

[15] Early modern physicians did not distinguish between syphilis and gonorrhea. Furthermore, the diagnostic term was the "French disease," not syphilis. It is important to avoid the problems of retrospective diagnoses by using contemporary disease categories. On this issue, see Jon Arrizabalaga, John Henderson, and Roger French, *The Great Pox: The French Disease in Renaissance Europe* (New Haven and London: Yale University Press, 1997), 1-3. Other useful accounts of the history of the French disease during this period include Anna Foa, "The New and the Old: The Spread of Syphilis (1494-1530)," in *Sex and Gender in Historical Perspective*, ed. Edward Muir and Guido Ruggiero (Baltimore: Johns Hopkins University Press, 1990); Bruce Thomas Buehrer, "Early Modern Syphilis," *Journal of the History of Sexuality* 1 (1990): 197-214; Claude Quétel, *History of Syphilis* (Baltimore: Johns Hopkins University Press, 1990); and Alfred W. Crosby, *The Columbian Exchange: Biological and Social Consequences of 1492* (Westport, CT: Greenwood Press, 1972), 122-164.

[16] Foa, "The New and the Old," 26-45.

[17] Laura J. McGough, "Quarantining Beauty: The French Disease in Early Modern Venice," in *Sins of the Flesh: Responding to Sexual Disease in Early Modern Europe*, ed. Kevin Siena (Toronto: Centre for Renaissance and Reformation Studies, 2005), 211-238.

[18] On the medical marketplace in England, see Kevin Siena, *Venereal Disease, Hospitals, and the Urban Poor: London's "Foul Wards" 1600-1800* (Rochester: University of Rochester Press, 2004); Kevin Siena, "The 'Foul Disease' and Privacy: The Effects of Venereal Disease and Patient Demand in the Medical Marketplace in Early Modern London," *Bulletin of the History of Medicine* 75 (2001): 199-224.

[19] Gianna Pomata, *Contracting a Cure: Patients, Healers, and the Law in Early Modern Bologna* (Baltimore: Johns Hopkins University Press, 1998).

[20] Laura J. McGough, "Demons or Nature? Witchcraft and the French Disease in Early Modern Venice," *Bulletin of the History of Medicine* 80 (2006): 219-246.

[21] Siena, *Venereal Disease, Hospitals, and the Urban Poor.*

[22] *Secreti Diversi & Miracolosi* (Venice: Alessandro Gardano, 1578), 43.

[23] Siena, *Venereal Disease, Hospitals, and the Urban Poor*, 214.

[24] McGough, "Quarantining Beauty."

[25] Winfried Schleiner, "Infection and Cure through Women: Renaissance Constructions of Syphilis," *Journal of Medieval and Renaissance Studies*, 24 (1994): 499-517.

[26] I discuss the examples of Angela Castellana and Camilla Savioni at length in "Demons or Nature? Witchcraft and the French Disease in Early Modern Venice." The editors of the *Bulletin* have given permission to reprint these examples.

[27] See Stuart Clark, *Thinking with Demons: the Idea of Witchcraft in Early Modern Europe* (Oxford: Clarendon Press, 1997); Guido Ruggiero, "The Strange Death of Margarita Marcellini: Male, Signs, and the Everyday World of Pre-Modern Medicine," *The American Historical Review* 106 (2001): 1-41.

[28] Archivio di Stato di Venezia (ASV), Sant'Uffizio, Busta 77, fasc. 21, contra Bellina Loredana, 1624.

[29] ASV, Sant'Uffizio, Busta 79, fasc. Savioni, Camilla.

[30] Louis F. Qualtiere and William W. E. Slights, "Contagion and Blame in Early Modern England: The Case of the French Pox," *Literature and Medicine* 22 (2003): 1-24; Jonathan Gil Harris, *Foreign Bodies and the Body Politic: Discourses of Social Pathology in Early Modern England* (Cambridge, UK: Cambridge University Press, 1998).

[31] Susan Sontag, *Illness as Metaphor* (New York: Vintage Books, 1977).

[32] Other common stigma-bearing illnesses are leprosy, mental illness and epilepsy. Veena Das discussed how stigma occurs across cultures and throughout history, albeit with culturally specific forms. See "Stigma, Contagion, Defect: Issues in the Anthropology of Public Health," http://www.stigmaconference.nih.gov/FinalDasPaper.htm.

[33] As Jo Stein argues, "The idea that stigma is the result of misinformation is, arguably, equivalent to the assumption that safer sex will result from knowledge of the routes of transmission. If only it were that simple." See "HIV/AIDS stigma: The latest dirty secret," *African Journal of AIDS Research* 2 (2003): 95-101, p. 96.

[34] Laura Nyblade et al., "Disentangling HIV and AIDS Stigma in Ethiopia, Tanzania, and Zambia," (Washington, DC: International Center for Research on Women, 2003), 20.

[35] Jessica Ogden and Laura Nyblade, *Common at Its Core: HIV-Related Stigma across Contexts* (Washington, DC: International Center for Research on Women, 2005), 20-21.

[36] Ann Sikwibele, Caroline Shonga and Carolyn Baylies, "AIDS in Kapulanga, Mongu: Poverty, Neglect and Gendered Patterns of Blame," in *AIDS, Sexuality and Gender in Africa: Collective Strategies and Struggles in Tanzania and Zambia*, ed.Carolyn Baylies and Janet Bujra (New York: Routledge, 2000), 60-76; Jessica Ogden and Laura Nyblade, "Common at Its Core," 24-5.

[37] Daniel Jordan Smith, "HIV/AIDS: Morality and Perceptions of Personal Risk in Nigeria," *Medical History* 22 (2003): 343-372, pp. 347-8.

[38] Jonas E. Okeagu, Joseph C. Okeagu, and Ademiluyi O. Adegoke, "The Impact on African Societies of the Standard Hypothesis that HIV/AIDS Originated in the Continent," *Journal of Third World Studies* XX (2003): 113-124.

[39] Allan Brandt, *No Magic Bullet: A Social History of Venereal Disease in the United States since 1880* (New York: Oxford University Press, 1987). See also Marilyn Hegarty, "Patriots, Prostitutes, Patriotutes: The Mobilization and Control of Female Sexuality in the United States during World War II" (Ph.D. dissertation, Ohio State University, 1998).

[40] Memo from Mr. Judson Hardy to Miss Lida Usilton, August 24, 1943. Record Group 90, Records of the Public Health Service, General Classified Records, Group X National Defense, 1940-46, 0425 Ven. Dis., 1940-44, Box 722, National Archives, College Park, MD.

[41] Hegarty, "Patriots, Prostitutes, Patriotutes."

[42] Leila Rupp, *Mobilizing Women for War: German and American Propaganda, 1939-1945* (Princeton: Princeton University Press, 1971); Susan Hartmann, *The Home Front and Beyond American Women in the 1940s* (Boston: Twayne Publishers, 1982).

[43] Conference of Preventive Medicine Officers, 158. Record Group 112, Office of the Surgeon General/Army World War II Administrative Records-7I.337, Box 694, National Archives, College Park, MD.

[44] L. J. McGough, S. J. Reynolds, T. C. Quinn, and J. M. Zenilman, "Which Patients First? Setting Priorities for Antiretroviral Therapy Where Resources Are Limited," *American Journal of Public Health* 95 (2005): 1173-1180.

[45] Paul Farmer, *Infections and Inequalities: The Modern Plagues* (Berkeley: University of California Press, 1999).

[46] A useful model could be the town hall meetings that have been used to develop health care priorities. These meetings are dialogues between local communities and public health officials, in which the public provides input into the establishment of priorities and provides feedback on official documents. See Norman Daniels and James E. Sabin, *Setting Limits Fairly: Can We Learn to Share Medical Resources?* (New York: Oxford University Press, 2002). Another model would be to borrow from the literature about conflict resolution and reconciliation, where historical examples form other cultures are used in order to show that conflict is a human problem, not restricted to particular ethnic groups. See Ervin Staub, Laurie Anne Pearlman, and Vachel Miller, "Healing the Roots of Genocide in Rwanda," *Peace Review* 15 (2003): 287-94.

[47] See for example Randall Packard and Paul Epstein, MD., "Epidemiologists, Social Scientists and Structure of Medical Research on AIDS in Africa," *Social Science and Medicine* 33 (1991): 771-794.

CHAPTER 7

Comments on Stigma and Behavior Change: Implications for HIV Prevention

JUDITH PORTER

According to UN AIDS, the most recent adjusted figures as of 2006 demonstrate that of the 38 million people in the world who are living with HIV infection, 25 million, or two-thirds, are in sub-Saharan Africa. In 2006, an estimated three million people in the region were newly infected. Women and girls in sub-Saharan Africa bear the brunt of the epidemic; they constitute 59% of adults living with AIDS. In seven southern African countries, the prevalence rate of HIV infection is 16% or more. In 2005, approximately 930,000 adults and children died of AIDS in sub-Saharan Africa. Treatment for AIDS is available to only a minority of those infected in this region. Only 17% of the 4.7 million people in need of anti-retroviral therapy receive it.[1] Prevention is of major importance in slowing the devastation the AIDS epidemic is causing in sub-Saharan Africa.

At the Bryn Mawr Medicine in Africa Workshop, I was the discussant of a panel with papers by Rachel Chapman, Julie Livingston, Laura McGough, and Susan Watkins, which have important implications for HIV prevention. Rachel Chapman's study ("Segredos da Casa: Managing the Social Risks of Reproduction in Central Mozambique") and Julie Livingston's paper ("Inside the Uterine Wall: Tswana Women's Sexuality and Nursing in a Changing Moral Landscape") do not appear in this volume.[2] However, to describe the contribution of this panel to the understanding of HIV prevention in Africa, it is necessary to review briefly their central themes, and to compare them to the issues raised by Laura McGough and Susan Watkins, whose papers are included in this book.

Chapman investigates perceptions of risk during pregnancy, how that risk is managed, and the structural factors that constrain these decisions in

Mozambique. Women view reproductive and pregnancy problems as caused by bad spirits, through witchcraft and sorcery (*feitiço*). Pregnancy is seen as a sign of good fortune and impending social wealth, so it has the potential to create ill will stemming from jealousy or power struggles among women in the family. Under these circumstances, *feitiço* is, as Chapman suggests, a "compelling discourse to interpret reproductive threats." The best way to avoid problems is to keep one's good fortune of pregnancy secret. This causal attribution of reproductive threats affects prenatal health-seeking behavior, leading to the use of traditional cures and folk treatments rather than modern medicine. Many women view health clinics as unable to address the true source of their reproductive risk. Witchcraft and sorcery are not only ways of interpreting reproductive risk during pregnancy, but are also based on power and resource inequalities and consequent stresses in social relationships. Thus, women's reproductive beliefs and practices are not due to lack of knowledge, but are expressions of wider structural problems.

Julie Livingston also stresses the relationship between reproductive and structural issues. In southeast Botswana, in the two decades after World War II, the symbolism of uteruses changed from generative to toxic and polluting. The change occurred as men's control over labor and sexuality shifted due to the male migrant labor system and women's labor migration. Female-headed families became prevalent because of long-term male absence. These factors resulted in an increase in extra- and pre-marital pregnancy, which was attributed to unchecked female autonomy. Sex meant the shared substance that tied lineage members together bodily, socially and economically (through either bride wealth or pregnancy compensation), so it concerned the lineage as much as the individual. The womb became a space where the toxic effects of women's autonomy were passed on as illness, threatening the health of the lineage and the community. Livingston's paper focuses on *mopakwane*, which links impairments in children to the mother's sexual behavior.

Although these two studies do not directly deal with AIDS, they present themes that McGough and Watkins also discuss in this volume. McGough suggests that illness becomes a metaphor of moral and cultural contagion. She interprets syphilis in 16th century Venice as symbolic of larger issues of social relationships and power, and she applies this analysis to the interpretation of AIDS origin and transmission in Mali. McGough, Livingston, and

Chapman all view the stigma of illness as embedded in broader patterns of power and social inequality. Watkins, in her research on prevention of HIV infection in Malawi, also views prevention as rooted in culture and structure. She stresses a communal rather than individual model of behavior change, and emphasizes the importance of social networks in the creation of indigenous strategies of AIDS prevention.

These four researchers interpret beliefs about disease origin, transmission, and risk not as lack of knowledge, but as expressions of structural issues and their articulation in culture. They challenge Western-based prevention models that tend to be individually oriented, based on rational choice (especially reliance on AIDS education), and recently in the case of the U.S., ideologically driven. These studies provide a deeper understanding of two basic issues in the prevention of HIV infection: combating stigma, and taking account of cultural understandings and structural realities.

The stigma of HIV infection must be addressed for HIV prevention to be effective. Reduction of stigma increases the willingness of an individual to be tested for HIV. It also helps protect the human rights of those who are infected. McGough and Livingston emphasize the role of metaphors in the way diseases are viewed. As Susan Sontag (1988), among others, has pointed out, disease is socially constructed.[3] McGough demonstrates Sontag's argument that illness throughout history has been described by metaphors and in turn is a metaphor for social and cultural tensions. Sexually transmitted diseases and medical conditions affecting women's bodies are especially used as metaphors for social and cultural strain. In Botswana, the view of women's wombs as toxic and polluting serves as a metaphor for the threat to men of greater female autonomy and the loss of social control over women's sexuality.[4] Family conflicts and women's social and economic marginalization are metaphorized as reproductive problems in Mozambique.[5] AIDS is used as a metaphor for social, economic, and political vulnerability and anxiety about Western post-colonial influence in Africa (McGough). Metaphors may not only symbolize social strain but also reinforce the stigma of particular medical conditions.

McGough points out that stigma is linked to broader patterns of social inequality. The marginalization and disempowerment of women, as well as changes in gender roles related to economic and other stresses, may reinforce the stigma of disease. AIDS thus becomes a ready metaphor for social structural dislocation and strain as well as for power inequality and vulnerability. Livingston does not directly address AIDS; she describes senyega in Lesotho. The symptoms of senyega in children (weight loss, severe diarrhea, failure to thrive) are also symptoms of pediatric AIDS. Since senyega in children is attributed to promiscuity of the mother, it will be interesting to see if this cultural attribution reinforces AIDS metaphors and stigma. Since disease is utilized as a metaphor of social and cultural strains, the stigma of AIDS cannot be eliminated simply by presenting information on AIDS prevention or by distributing condoms without addressing these structural strains and inequalities.

AIDS prevention depends not only on addressing stigma and its structural roots but also on changing behavior. Watkins points out that both risk perception and cultural understandings of sexuality are critical factors in the prevention of HIV infection. Rather than focusing on the efficacy of externally imposed prevention programs, she views the cultural perceptions of peer networks in Malawi as primary sources of behavior change. The networks themselves, based on their cultural understandings of AIDS, play an important role in innovating strategies for modifying HIV risk behavior. Locally formulated prevention strategies are based not only on epidemiological information and evidence of AIDS deaths, but also on the social construction of sexuality and HIV risk. She views indigenous sources of behavior change as a result of confluence of these factors. Chapman also stresses the importance of cultural interpretation in behavior change in her analysis of the utilization of modern health-seeking strategies among pregnant women in Mozambique

In the harm reduction model, successful AIDS prevention is viewed as any reduction in the risk of contracting HIV rather than as the elimination of risk. Watkins investigates indigenous strategies for reducing the risk of HIV infection. These strategies include a reliance on "born again" or spirit-type religions that create a defense against evil forces and reinforce marital fidelity. They also include a focus not on strict fidelity but on compromises such as the reduction in number of partners, more careful selection, and use of condoms primarily with culturally defined risky partners. These strategies lower to some extent but do not eliminate the chance of being infected. They may be more effective in the aggregate than for a particular individual since they reduce the number of infections in sexual networks and thus lower the probability of HIV transmission. Watkins sees women as actors in prevention, through attempts to persuade a spouse to be faithful or to divorce her if she suspects he is infected. She also stresses the importance of peer norms in the prevention of HIV. She treats these innovative local strategies as positive forces for HIV/AIDS prevention, rather than viewing them in judgmental terms or as barriers to behavior change.

Watkins makes the important point that people in Malawi are not isolated automatons or passive victims. Based on their social context and cultural understandings, they develop their own creative prevention strategies and compromises. Her study suggests that for prevention models to be successful, locally generated prevention strategies and existing cultural understandings must be taken into account. Local cultural understandings may also be counterproductive in HIV prevention. Chapman, for instance, describes spirit wives in Mozambique who are ritually married to avenging spirits but may be at high risk of contracting HIV through the expectation that they have sex with multiple partners. However, local understandings of sexuality and disease, regardless of their efficacy as HIV prevention strategies, must be considered when formulating any prevention campaign.

These studies suggest a number of important implications for AIDS prevention. First, prevention strategies need to focus not just on individual AIDS prevention interventions, as most Western models do, but on strategies that involve social and community networks and their cultural understandings of the disease. Second, prevention strategies need to take into account not just the level of community networks but also the macro-social level. Economic and gender inequalities are the basis of the AIDS epidemic and need to be addressed as major components of prevention, especially the social and economic empowerment of women. As Chapman demonstrates, to understand why modern health seeking strategies and illness-prevention behavior may not be automatically adopted, one needs to understand both the role of gender and of economic marginalization in risk perception and the cultural understanding of illness. Third, people must be viewed as actors, not simply as victims; they negotiate their own prevention strategies when possible. This does not contradict the more macro-structural stress on sources of stigma. Prevention strategies are negotiated within a local context bounded by larger cultural metaphors that are based on cultural and structural strain. This indicates once again the necessity of working on both micro and macro levels to prevent AIDS.

The works discussed here provide a critique of the ABC (Abstinence, Be faithful, use Condoms) strategy that has been the focus of AIDS prevention in Uganda. They suggest that this tactic is not uniformly applicable and may work for some subgroups better than others; that sexual behavior change should be generated by addressing cultural understandings of sexuality; and that condoms are needed not only for high risk *groups* like sex workers (as the Bush administration currently stresses in its African AIDS initiative) but can and should be initially introduced for what is perceived as high risk *behavior* for *all* members of society. The research presented in these papers explains the findings of recent studies that "Abstinence" and "Be faithful" have not been the primary sources of reducing the prevalence of AIDS in Uganda; instead, the availability of condoms and the high death rate have been the major factors.[6]

The stress on cultural understandings and innovation by local peer groups does not deny the importance of government support of AIDS prevention. In fact, the role of government in the de-stigmatization of AIDS and protection of human rights is crucial for the prevention of HIV disease. South Africa, which has the second largest number of HIV infections of any country, shows the devastating effects of lack of government support as far as prevention is concerned. The works by McGough, Livingston, Watkins, and Chapman suggest, either directly or indirectly, that prevention strategies must be sensitive to local cultural understandings and structural inequalities to be effective. AIDS prevention programs cannot be successful if they are judgmental, ideologically based, individually oriented models imposed from outside the society. The implications for AIDS prevention presented in these papers apply as much to high-risk communities in the U.S. as they do to the African societies described by these four researchers.

Notes

[1] UN AIDS, *2006 Report on the Global AIDS Epidemic, Executive Summary* (Geneva, Switzerland: UN AIDS, 2006), 1-23.

[2] The papers by Chapman and Livingston are published elsewhere. See Rachel Chapman, "Segredos da Casa: Social Risks and Reproductive Threats in Central Mozambique," *Medical Anthropology Quarterly* 20 (2006): 487-515; and Julie Livingston, *Debility and Moral Imagination in Botswana* (Bloomington: Indiana University Press, 2005).

[3] Susan Sontag, *AIDS and Its Metaphors* (New York: Farrar, Strauss, and Giroux, 1988).

[4] Livingston, *Debility and Moral Imagination in Botswana.*

[5] Chapman, "Segredos da Casa."

[6]M. J. Wawer, R. Gray, D. Serwadda, et al, "Declines in HIV Prevalence in Uganda: Not as Simple as ABC" (presentation at the 12th Conference on Retroviruses and Opportunistic Infection, Boston, Massachusetts, February 22-25, 2005).

CHAPTER 8

Malaria and the Peopling of Early Tropical Africa[1]

JAMES L. A. WEBB, JR.

The first chapters in human prehistory are the story of early humanity in tropical Africa. Over long epochs of foraging, our ancestors gradually developed tools, adapted to new environments, and created more complex material culture. The internal dynamics of the early epochs of the human past in tropical Africa, however, have remained relatively obscure. By contrast, the rapid advances of humanity in regions outside of tropical Africa during the extended Neolithic agricultural revolution are generally agreed to mark a revolutionary break with the early epochs. For this reason, it is customary for world historians, after acknowledging a long history of human foraging, to begin the teaching of world history with the agrarian era, some ten or eleven thousand years ago.[2]

This essay synthesizes research findings in the fields of microbiology, archaeology, and archaeobotany to explore the significance of malaria on the peopling of early tropical Africa, before the Common Era. Malaria emerged as a human disease in tropical Africa, and over the long run of humankind on earth, it has likely killed more Africans than any other disease. This essay advances evidence that human genetic responses to malarial infections in early tropical Africa constitute the earliest known chapters in the human experience with infectious disease, revising the idea that the first accommodations to infectious disease environments took place in the agricultural settlements in the fertile river basins of northern Africa and southern and eastern Eurasia. It also advances a new interpretation of the colonization of much of tropical Africa during the fifth to first millennia B.C.E. demographic processes known as the "Bantu expansions." It contends that human accommodations to endemic malarial infections – in conjunction with the practice of yam and plantain vegeculture – resulted in an "immunological gradient" between rainforest villagers and foragers that played a major role in the expansion of Bantu-speaking peoples. This interpretation revises older interpretations that have stressed the role of iron making and political violence and supplements newer interpretations that have focused on cultural and linguistic evidence. This synthesis argues against the significance of diffusionist influences and for a more integrated theory of the peopling of early tropical Africa.

Tropical Africa and Human Disease History

In 1976, William H. McNeill published *Plagues and Peoples*, a highly influential synthesis of the history of human disease. In it the author argued that the disease environment of tropical Africa held a special significance for understanding early human history. The tropical African disease environment was extremely difficult, owing to the sheer variety of parasites that preyed upon human beings and of vector-borne diseases to which human beings were subject. Indeed, the first great advance in human health was the successful exodus of some human pioneers from tropical Africa. Outside of the African tropics, human emigrants discovered that they had left the ecological zones in which some of the most virulent vector-borne diseases were endemic and that as a result their disease burden was lighter. This improvement in health or, put differently, this increase in reproductive fitness, in turn led to more rapid population growth and ultimately to the establishment of settled communities, marking the most important transition – the agricultural revolution – in the long prehistory of humankind.[3]

For McNeill, subsequent major early developments in the history of humankind's relation to infectious disease thus took place outside of humid tropical Africa, with the growth of agricultural settlements in the fertile river basins of northern Africa (the Nile) and elsewhere around the southern and eastern reaches of Eurasia (Tigris-Euphrates, Indus, Yangtze, and Yellow Rivers). In these river basins, human beings began to experiment with the domestication of herd animals, and the close proximity of dense-settled human populations with herd animals allowed for some of the pathogens of herd animals to adapt to human beings. A series of major, infectious, nontropical zoonoses such as chickenpox, smallpox, influenza, and measles emerged as diseases of human beings in this manner. Other infectious diseases, both bacterial and viral, that were either waterborne or transmitted by fecal-oral contamination likewise emerged in the centers of human settlement, where populations were sufficiently dense to support "crowd diseases." The consequences of this onslaught of infectious disease were momentous. The river basin populations suffered greatly but eventually developed limited immunities, and when the disease-experienced populations made contact with non-disease-experienced populations, the result was demographic shock (and sometimes collapse), with high rates of mortality and morbidity, among non-disease-experienced populations.[4]

Historians of Africa have credited the difficult disease environment of tropical Africa with a vital role in shaping the history of African civilizations. In a broad sense, the disease environment has been understood as a core challenge to the establishment of African civilizations.[5] The difficult disease environment of tropical Africa is also held to have isolated tropical Africa, to some degree, from broader contacts with the wider world. It limited contacts between North Africa and sub-Saharan Africa and influenced the interactions between pastoral nomadic peoples and agricultural peoples in the sahel.[6] It raised the health costs of both Atlantic and Indian Ocean maritime contacts and thereby constrained the nature and extent of those interactions. The tropical African disease barrier is generally accepted as the principal reason why Africa was not colonized by Europeans during the same era as the Americas and why the long centuries of the Atlantic slave trade along the western coast of Africa took place between European traders and independent African states.[7] Until very recently, however, there was little evidence to suggest that there were older disease processes that shaped earlier periods of the African past.

The Genomes of the Malarial Parasites

Over the past several years, microbiologists have decoded the genomes for two of the principal malarial parasites that have played such an enormous role in world history: *Plasmodium vivax* and *Plasmodium falciparum*.[8] In their recent article in *Clinical Microbiology Reviews* (2002), Richard Carter and Kamimi N. Mendis have skillfully assayed the microbiological research literature and other natural science and historical literatures on malaria to produce a major synthesis on the "Evolutionary and Historical Aspects of the Burden of Malaria."[9]

Plasmodium vivax

The genetic molecular evidence for vivax indicates that it is very ancient and that it diverged from an earlier malarial parasite that infected both apes and protohuman beings approximately two to three million years ago. It seems likely that vivax originated in Africa because of the strikingly broad and concentrated distribution of the genetic mutation known as red blood cell Duffy antigen negativity (hereafter "Duffy negativity") in contemporary West and Central African populations.[10] This genetic mutation is found on an antigen receptor on the hemoglobin molecule that is normally invaded by the vivax parasite. Duffy negativity renders the individual with this mutation unable to contract vivax malaria.[11]

When did this mutation arise? The molecular genetic evidence indicates that vivax diverged from a parasite of Old World monkeys, *Plasmodium cynomologi*, approximately two to three million years ago. It thereafter developed into a scourge of the hominids. It is not possible to estimate the extent of the disease burden that vivax imposed in earliest Africa – or even during the career of *Homo sapiens* over the last few hundred thousand years – because of the multitude of ecological variables that are involved in malaria transmission and the fact that these vary over space and time. It is certain, however, that this disease burden increased over time. Powerful evidence of this increasing burden can be inferred from the fact that the mosquitoes that are the principal vectors for malaria on the African continent, *Anopheles gambiae* and *Anopheles funestus*, developed a marked preference for human blood – rather than animal or bird blood – and became the most efficient of the world's malaria-transmitting, anopheline vectors.

It is not possible to estimate the morbidity or mortality costs imposed by the increasing malarial burden. It is possible, however, and perhaps even likely, that the comparatively low levels of virulence that are documented today in a variety of vivax malaria environments – with mortality usually in the range of 1 to 2 percent, with exceptional mortality up to 5 percent – are lower than they were in earlier epochs. This would be in keeping with a general pattern of the attenuation of virulence when diseases of the humid tropics are transferred to other environments that are either less humid or less warm (or both). In these conditions, infectious agents often make accommodations to facilitate their transmission under less favorable conditions.[12]

And there are other uncertainties that cloud even the big picture of

Duffy negativity. It is not possible to determine where the genetic variation arose or if it arose independently in more than one population. And yet at some point after the migrations of modern human beings out of tropical Africa – a process that is generally held to have taken place during the period 100,000-50,000 B.P. and perhaps 70,000-50,000 B.P.[13] – our early ancestors apparently succeeded largely in throwing off the burden of vivax malaria that would later torment populations elsewhere around the planet.[14] An extraordinary 97 percent of West and Central African populations today carry the mutation for Duffy negativity and thus are physically unable to contract vivax malaria. This genetic adaptation has come without any negative health consequences, unlike other genetic adaptations that human beings have undergone in response to malarial infection.[15]

The Spread of Duffy Negativity

What forces might have proved conducive to this genetic adaptation? And when, approximately, did this genetic adaptation become widespread? There is no direct evidence that bears on these questions, and all attempts to answer them proceed from logical inference. A common view among microbiologists is that Duffy negativity likely occurred at the very end of the long period 97,200-6500 B.P. There are two strands of reasoning. One stresses the importance of climate change as a precursor to the emergence of the "Neolithic agricultural revolution." In this view, climate change – the rapid warming of the planet at the end of the last glacial period – was responsible for more mosquitoes and thus an increase in the malarial burden.[16] This increased burden was unstable, and the burden was further amplified when the climate began to warm. This warming was coincident with the beginnings of agriculture in tropical Africa, stimulated by the arrival of seeds and new technologies from the early river basin civilizations. According to this interpretation, the arrival of the "Neolithic agricultural revolution" provoked a vigorous biological response – progress toward the near fixation in the West and Central African populations of Duffy negativity – that blunted the force of vivax malaria.[17] According to this view of world history, human populations in humid tropical Africa did not begin to enjoy an increase in their rates of population growth and cultural development until the introduction of new seeds and technologies that emerged from the river basin civilizations and then diffused south.[18]

From the standpoint of recent Africanist archaeology, this interpretation of the history of Duffy negativity is somewhat problematic. If the selective fixation of Duffy negativity took place in the period beginning ca. 3000-2000 B.C.E., this adaptive genetic mutation would have required a high level of integration among disparate populations during a relatively brief period of several thousand years in order to be transmitted extensively throughout West and Central African populations to produce the near universal present-day distribution. This high level of integration is not suggested by cultural or linguistic studies.

The archaeological record does, however, suggest other possibilities for understanding the emergence and fixation of Duffy negativity that are consonant with a new appreciation of Africa's role in early human history. In recent years, Africanist archaeologists have done much to revise the chronologies of human evolution that were developed based on the European archaeological record, in light of the longer African archaeological sequences. In the broadest sense, it is now clear that not only did *Homo sapiens* emerge in Africa, but that very early processes of human cultural evolution took place in tropical Africa.

The findings of Africanist archaeologists have overturned the "human revolution" model of development that held that "modern" behavior of human beings gained first expression in Europe in a burst of evolutionary change. Instead, the Africanist findings have located the origins of "modern" human behavior where one might have suspected – in Africa – and revised the basic chronology of early human history. The discovery of an early "middle Stone Age worked bone industry" – thought to represent large-scale seasonal fishing expeditions that would have necessitated seasonal settlement – located the early origins of complex thinking and behavior necessary for major cultural changes in east-central Africa rather than in Europe. This discovery also pushed back the temporal horizon of these cultural changes from ca. 35,000 B.P. to ca. 89,000 B.P.[19] Indeed, it now appears that the transition from the middle Stone Age to the late Stone Age in tropical Africa was an extremely gradual process that took place over perhaps two hundred thousand years.

These new interpretations of the African archaeological evidence thus argue for an African origin of new human cultural behaviors that arose at varying times and places across the African continent, and that these behaviors were exported with the African migrants who left to populate other regions of Eurasia. The archaeological record of these cultural achievements, although interrupted during glacial maxima in some parts of Africa such as the Sahara and the interior of Cape Province in South Africa, are sufficiently numerous in other African biomes, including the expanses of steppe, savanna, and woodland, to support the idea of the continuous presence of probably widely dispersed human populations across these diverse environments.[20]

Africanist archaeologists have also documented the intensification of African cultural practices after about 50,000 B.P. – including novel technologies such as new projectiles that increased the productivity of hunting and new fishing methods that allowed for the more efficient exploitation of a vast resource – which meant that the newly available technologies could support larger populations in a given territory. Moreover, these technologies apparently allowed for human groups to expand into new habitats, such as the tropical forest.[21] For the study of early malaria, the cumulative significance of these archaeological findings is that they make the point that human communities living in tropical Africa did not wait until the arrival of a Neolithic "development package" ca. 3000 B.C.E. to expand their exploitation of new environments – including those that were ideal for the transmission of malarial infections.

The very early patterns of seasonal migration and riverbank settlement – tens of thousands of years before the last glacial maximum – would have provided ideal conditions for seasonal – and thus, unstable – malarial infection. In one of the ironies of malarial infection, it is the lower levels of infection (as compared to stable endemic malaria among settled communities) that create very dangerous patterns of transmission – what is known as unstable malaria.[22] Today, vivax malaria in regions outside of Africa is associated with low levels of mortality (under 5 percent, and often in the range of 1 to 2 percent); this is thought to result from the ancient spread of vivax malaria to nontropical-African regions in which stable rates of transmission produced limited immunity through repeated infection. According to this line of argument, unstable conditions in early Africa – with higher attendant mortality – would have produced selection pressures that strongly favored the spread of Duffy negativity.[23] The upshot is that it is no longer necessary to propose a dramatic "malaria revolution" in early tropical Africa that is a product of the introduction of a "Neolithic agricultural revolution," or to link the refractoriness to vivax malaria exclusively to a cycle of climate change. It appears far more likely that the refractoriness to vivax malaria emerged across the long process of human cultural evolution, in which human beings entered into new biomes and practiced seasonal settlement over a period of many tens of thousands of years.

This gradualist model of the spread of Duffy negativity is necessarily speculative. Its strengths are (1) that it is consonant with the microbiologists' broad time estimate for the emergence of Duffy negativity and (2) that it fits well with the archaeologists' interpretations of their data. The implications of the gradualist model are that, on the basis of available evidence, human refractoriness to vivax malaria as a result of Duffy negativity appears to be the very earliest known chapter in human beings' genetic adaptation to vector-borne infectious disease and, indeed, the very earliest known chapter in humanity's long struggle with parasitic disease. This genetic adaptation appears to have occurred well before Eurasian populations domesticated livestock and thereby gained limited immunities to the parasites that were attached to the domesticated animals of the Eurasian steppe – the horse, cow, goat, sheep, camel, and yak – or, for that matter, the donkey of the Nilotic steppe.[24]

The demographic consequence of the emergence of Duffy negativity was likely significant. Its fixation reduced the disease burden for the communities who inherited the mutation and contributed thereby to an increase in their population. Ongoing population growth was further facilitated by the new technologies and strategies that human communities developed in the post-50,000 B.P. period. Thus, on this basis alone, all other things being equal, it seems probable that an accelerated process of population growth among some populations in sub-Saharan Africa began to occur in an early period – well before the arrival of seeds and new technologies from the early river basin civilizations. It is likely that Duffy negativity became even more widely expressed during the processes of more intensive rainforest exploitation that occurred in more recent millennia and that are discussed later in this essay.

Plasmodium falciparum

The genetic molecular evidence concerning the emergence of modern *Plasmodium falciparum* is ambiguous, and microbiologists are not agreed on its interpretation. On the one hand, molecular analysis has shown that an ancestral parasite of simian falciparum malaria diverged from the even older parasite of bird malaria approximately 130 million years ago, and the molecular analysis strongly suggests that modern human falciparum malaria diverged from an ancestral form that was common to both apes and protohumans approximately 4 to 10 million years ago, very roughly coincident with the epoch during which the humanoid line diverged from the line of the African great apes.[25]   But another part of the parasite genome suggests a more recent development. One line of investigation has suggested that the modern form of falciparum diverged from a protofalciparum parasite very recently, that is, only in the period 8000-3000 B.C.E.[26] And, most recently, a comparison of mitochondrial genome sequences has found a major stepwise growth in the parasite population (a proxy for the increased incidence of human infection) in the period 13,000-8000 B.C.E.[27] These findings indicate that human beings in Africa experienced a marked increase in *P. falciparum* infections many millennia before the earliest (ca. 3000 B.C.E.) adoption of the package of Neolithic tools and seed agriculture by tropical African communities.[28]   The molecular evidence suggests that large-scale falciparum infections may have occurred tens of thousands of years later than vivax infections. One likely reason can be found in differences in life cycles of the plasmodia: chains of vivax infection are easier to sustain among hunters and gatherers and in groups that practice seasonal settlement because vivax parasites have a period of incubation in their life cycle that takes place in the human liver and can last for six to nine months. After incubation in the liver, vivax malaria can relapse – for up to as long as three years after the initial infection. Thus, vivax parasites could travel with the seasonal settler back into the rainforest or woodland or savanna, and carriers would remain able to infect mosquitoes and continue the chain long after leaving the settlement site. By contrast, falciparum sufferers remained infectious for a far shorter period of time. For this reason, the transmission of falciparum malaria is far more dependent upon continuous high host density.[29]

The human genetic accommodations to falciparum infections were also fraught with difficulties. Members of human communities who suffered assaults from falciparum parasites in tropical Africa came to carry a genetic mutation of the hemoglobin molecule known as sickle cell hemoglobin, or hemoglobin S. In some tropical African communities today, up to 25 or 30 percent of the population have inherited the sickle cell gene from one of their parents and a normal hemoglobin gene from the other parent and are thus heterozygous for the mutation. Children who are heterozygous for the sickle cell gene have only one-tenth the risk of death from falciparum as do those who are homozygous for the normal hemoglobin gene.[30] There is, however, a decided downside to the sickle cell. Those carriers who inherit the gene from both parents and thus are homozygous for sickle cell develop sickle cell anemia. They suffer an early death, before the age of reproduction. The sickle cell mutation thus conveys both costs and benefits to the human communities in which it becomes established. In genetic terms, the distribution of the sickle cell is thought to increase to the point where the aggregate survival advantages for heterozygous carriers balance the costs of sickle cell anemia to these communities. At this point it is considered to be in equilibrium, as a "balanced polymorphism."[31]

Early Processes of Rainforest Exploitation

Researchers in the fields of agronomy and archaeobotany have developed new understandings of early human exploitation of the African tropical rainforest environments. Their findings have complicated the simple and familiar model of the development of human societies that postulated that early (modern) human groups in tropical Africa were hunters, gatherers, and fishers; that after the introduction of seed agriculture, human groups settled and multiplied more rapidly; and that thereafter, human societies became complex. Recent research in archaeology and historical linguistics has upended a long-standing view that the introduction of agriculture from the early river basin societies triggered a revolutionary advance in tropical African societies. This older view can be thought of as the "diffusionist" model of development.

This diffusionist model has come under challenge from Africanist scholars who have investigated human development in humid tropical Africa in the late Stone Age. One dimension of their challenge is temporal: it involves a revision of our understanding of the era in which human groups began to exploit more fully the rainforest resources. The history of the oil palm (*Elaeis guineensis* Jacq.) and the West African white and yellow Guinea yams (*Dioscoreae cayenensis* and *D. rotundata*, respectively), all of which occurred naturally in the West African transitional biome between the woodlands and the forest, have been of particular research interest.[32]

The oil palm today is found in both West and West Central Africa. Specialists think that the occurrence of the oil palm is older in West Africa than in West Central Africa, and some hold that human beings probably played a role in its introduction and expansion into the rainforests of West Central Africa early in the Holocene period (7000-2500 B.C.E.). By the late Holocene it had become a common element in the subsistence economy in both West and West Central Africa. According to the archaeobotanist M. A. Sowunmi, it is likely that the human use of fire in rainforest clearings prevented the regrowth of forest trees in the openings and thus brought about an anthropogenically enhanced expansion of the natural oil palm stands. The oil palm, from which edible oils (both palm kernel oil and palm oil) can be extracted and which can be tapped for toddy to make wine, is one of the most economically useful plants in West and West Central Africa.[33] This interpretation of the archaeobotanical evidence for the expansion of the oil palm holds that it is a proxy for the increased human presence in and exploitation of the rainforest biome.[34]

The question of the cultivation origins of the white and yellow Guinea yams, distinguished by their high caloric yields, has attracted the attention of researchers since the 1960s. In publications during the 1960s and 1970s, the preeminent scholar of West African yams, D. G. Coursey, advanced an evolutionary model of yam use that reached far back in time. He held that hunters and gatherers had exploited wild yams even before 60,000 B.P. and that in the period 45,000 to 15,000 B.P. the late Stone Age peoples had begun to develop ritual concepts and practices to protect the yam plants. According to Coursey, by 9000 B.C.E. these peoples had begun to develop a "protoculture" based on the replanting of selected wild plants.

In Coursey's model, a "diffusionist" impulse remained important. In his view, by 3000 to 2000 B.C.E. Neolithic grain cultivators, influenced by the agriculturalists of southwestern Eurasia, had moved south from the Middle Niger River valley, interacted with the "protoculturalists," and created yam cultivation. For Coursey, this yam culture began to spread deeper into the forest with the advent of iron working, around 500 B.C.E. The forest ecologies favored cultivation of the yam over grain crops, and yam growers could produce more calories and thus achieve numerical superiority over grain farmers and create complex culture systems.[35]

The concept of protocultivation has itself been revised since the time of Coursey's pioneering work. Recent scholarship has argued for early African yam practices that were highly productive but were not a stepping-stone on the path to cultivation. Edmond Dounias has termed this "paracultivation" to distinguish it from the evolutionistically weighted term "protocultivation." In essence, paracultivation consists of the voluntary reburial of the wild yam head after tuber harvesting. The plant is thereby maintained in its original environment.[36] These practices apparently advanced the "ennoblement" of the guinea yams – that is, the genetic selection of the better yams to harvest and propagate that resulted in harvestable tubers that were far superior for comestible purposes to those produced by wild plants.

Linguists have also developed historical evidence of early yam cultivation. In the 1980s, the linguist Christopher Ehret judged that the words for "cultivation" and "yam" in proto-Niger-Congo date back to at least 8000 B.C.E. Recently, Ehret has synthesized a wealth of archaeological evidence and located the invention of "West African planting agriculture" by at least 8000 B.C.E. – thousands of years before the arrival of Neolithic seeds and agricultural techniques from the Fertile Crescent or before the emergence of the complex societies that arose in the middle valley of the Niger.[37] These new understandings of early Holocene exploitation of the rainforest edges and rainforest openings for yam paracultivation and then yam cultivation delink further the African historical experience from the diffusionist model that stressed the adoption of the "Neolithic agricultural revolution" by hunters and gatherers in tropical Africa.

An Immunological Gradient in Tropical Africa

Yam paracultivation and then yam cultivation took place in cleared woodlands near the rainforests or in rainforest openings. These microenvironments were created through the use of fire and the stone ax – and beginning in the first millennium B.C.E., the iron ax. There were direct epidemiological implications. The fire-cleared openings in woodland and rainforest were the ideal environments for the gambiae and funestus mosquitoes to breed in. (These mosquitoes do not breed in swamps or full rainforests.) The cultivation of yams entailed lengthier residence and work in sites conducive to anopheline mosquito breeding, and thus encounters with falciparum malaria would have intensified with the shift from paracultivation to cultivation. It seems likely that at this era the increasing burden of falciparum parasites

– with many first attacks fatal and others debilitating – began to select for a genetic mutation to mitigate the damage.[38]

Within the early tropical woodland and rainforest settlements, new disease dynamics became established. When yam paracultivators became yam cultivators and remained near their plantings, this created an environment of continual malarial infection, with paradoxical consequences. Individuals who survive the initial bouts of falciparum malaria and live in environments of endemic infection with high parasite loads develop short-term partial immunities that greatly reduce suffering from the disease. In this respect, after the initial onslaught of falciparum malaria, the survivors are much safer if they continue to live in a settlement of continuous stable infection. When individuals leave, for periods of even less than one year, their immunities deteriorate.

The world of the early yam-growing tropical African village was thus, in epidemiological terms, a different disease world from the rainforest that surrounded it. When hunters and gatherers made even brief contact with villages of stable falciparum infection – yet where the villagers themselves appeared to be in good health – these contacts produced sharply elevated mortality and morbidity among hunters and gatherers, who were at ongoing risk for death and debilitation at successive contacts. Thus, the establishment of permanent settlements in tropical Africa created an "immunological gradient" that shifted steeply from villagers to hunters and gatherers in the rainforests and woodlands around them.

Tropical Vegecultural Frontiers

From the woodlands of West Africa, pioneers extended the practice of vegeculture, centered on yam cultivation, deep into the rainforests. There were two major frontiers of this multiregional, vegecultural expansion. One was within West Africa itself. The West African speakers of languages of the "West Atlantic" grouping of the Niger-Congo language family moved south from the savanna and woodlands into the rainforest belt above the Gulf of Guinea. These rainforests were not entirely unfamiliar to them, and indeed there were no autochthonous peoples who spoke languages from a different language grouping in the West African rainforests.[39] From the point of view of historical linguistics, these movements have attracted relatively little scholarly attention.

A second frontier of expansion was initiated from the border of what is today Nigeria and Cameroon. From this region, Bantu speakers spread across tropical Africa to the south and east, into West Central and East Africa. They encountered hunters and gatherers who were Batwa speakers, and over a period of a few thousand years, in two great migrations (5000-4000 B.C.E. and 1500-500 B.C.E.), the Bantu speakers spread their languages over the vast expanse of equatorial Africa and much of eastern Africa. Because of the relatively recent periods in which these migrations took place and the phenomenal extension of the Bantu language zone, the Bantu speakers' phases of expansion have attracted the attention of scholars from a variety of disciplines.[40]

Recently, Kairn Klieman has brilliantly reconceptualized the relationship between Bantu-speaking villagers and Batwa-speaking peoples ("Pygmies"). She argues from cultural and linguistic evidence that the relationship between Bantu-speaking immigrants and Batwa-speaking hunting and gathering authochthons that began with the first Bantu migration (5000-4000 B.C.E.) was profoundly changed with the introduction of the banana / plantain complex and iron working during the second Bantu expansion, in the late Stone to Metal Age (1500-500 B.C.E.).[41]

Probably during the end of the second millennium B.C.E. or the first half of the first millennium B.C.E., the plantain / banana complex spread west from eastern Africa into the central equatorial rainforests.[42] There it likely took over the role of the staple food.[43] The plantain / banana complex, along with yam cultivation and, by this late date, some use of seed agriculture, provided a robust basis for village settlement. In the same ways that the yam and oil palm played important roles in the opening of the rainforests during the late Holocene, in later millennia tropical Africans widely adopted the plantain / banana complex and incorporated it into the heart of their rainforest village economies.

Over the course of these "Bantu" migrations, and particularly following the adoption of the banana / plantain complex, rainforest villagers were able to establish larger permanent settlements in the rainforests that became centers of falciparum infection.[44] This disease process must have been one of the major factors that led to the replacement of non-Bantu-speaking peoples with Bantu-speaking peoples over vast areas of the continent in a very slow process that unfolded over many centuries.[45] Falciparum malaria would have dramatically reduced the numbers of all peoples who visited the village zones of stable malaria, much as it dramatically killed European visitors millennia later during the years of the Atlantic slave trade, the era of the "white man's grave."

Historians have hitherto sought explanations for the expansion of the Bantu speakers in other material processes, such as the adoption of yam cultivation (which yields large numbers of calories and would have contributed to population growth) and the adoption of new iron technologies. The pairing of yams and iron, however, has been criticized on the basis that iron tools are not necessary for yam cultivation. (Wooden digging sticks are admirably suited to the work.) Others have held that in the Bantu migrations, the principal use of iron was for weaponry, strengthening the ability of the Bantu speakers to dominate in war.[46] This argument is greatly weakened by the lack of any archaeological or linguistic evidence of such warfare.

A more plausible interpretation emerges from the consideration of the processes of rainforest exploitation and the dynamics of falciparum infection. The expansion of the zone of Bantu language speakers appears to be based upon the demographic advantages of high-yielding yam and plantain / banana cultivation, in conjunction with a tropical falciparum malarial "immunological gradient." In this light, the processes of the Bantu expansions are direct analogues to the expansions of the disease-experienced peoples of early village Eurasia.[47] The contemporary distribution of sickle cell mutations in West and Central Africa bears eloquent witness to the end results of these early processes. Today, sickle cell mutations occur in two major independent groups identified on the basis of the location on the gene of the hemoglobin mutation: 7.6-kb fragment and 13-kb fragment. The first is found in Central Africa in the Zaire basin. The second is found in the Niger delta region. A third independent origin of sickle cell mutation, which is less severe in its consequences for homozygous individuals, is centered in Sierra Leone.[48]

The map in Figure 8.1 displays the spatial distribution of the three independent mutations of the sickle cell mutations. As Stuart Edelstein, one of the leading authorities on sickle cell, has argued, both the 13-kb and 7.6-kb fragments offer the same protection against falciparum malaria for those heterozygous for the mutations and the same costs for those who are homozygous. The mutations could not have arisen prior to the Bantu expansions, otherwise, the 7.6-kb mutation, to establish itself so prominently, would have had to confer a decisive advantage over the 13-kb mutation, which it does not. Edelstein estimated that these mutations arose independently in recent millennia, probably during the first millennium B.C.E. and/or the first millennium C.E.[49] This estimate would be roughly coincident with or follow the full adoption of the plantain / banana complex. Thus, sickle cell, even if now widely distributed, appears to have emerged only in the final centuries of, or even in the aftermath of, the second Bantu expansion.

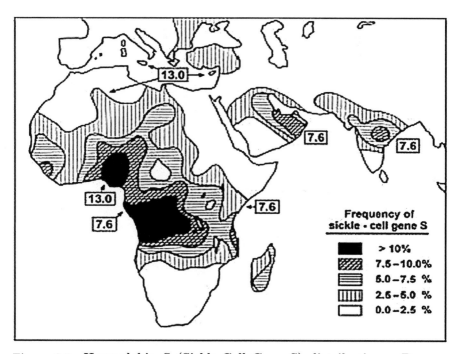

Figure 8.1: Hemoglobin S (Sickle-Cell Gene S) distributions. Reproduced from Stuart J. Edelstein, *The Sickled Cell: From Myths to Molecules* (Cambridge, Mass.: Harvard University Press, 1986), fig. 7.3, p. 149 with permission from Harvard University Press. (Adapted from Yuet Wai Kan and Andree M. Dozy, "Evolution of the Hemoglobin S and C Genes in World Populations," *Science*, n.s. 209, no. 4454 [1980], 388-391. Copyright 1980 by the AAAS.)

Conclusion

This essay examines microbiologists' evidence for the genomes for vivax and falciparum malaria as means to explore demographic processes in early tropical Africa that predate the food revolutions of the early river basin civilizations. It suggests that there were very early processes of growth and change in tropical Africa that unfolded independently from the historical processes that took place in the great river basin civilizations, including that of the Middle Niger. The molecular biological evidence suggests that malaria was a principal constraint to population growth in tropical Africa and that this demographic challenge existed well before the establishment of permanently settled communities. The challenge of vivax malaria apparently began to be met by the emergence of Duffy negativity long before the rise of the river basin civilizations. Refractoriness to vivax meant *ipso facto* an enhanced possibility of demographic growth. The development of new fishing and hunting technologies after 50,000 B.P. increased the ease with which human groups harvested food and thereby contributed to population growth. Indeed, it is possible that this population pressure was in part responsible for the increasing forays into the forests and the early transition from yam gathering to paracultivation and then to cultivation.[50] In these contexts, Duffy negativity became more widely expressed in tropical African populations.

The demographic challenge created by falciparum malaria is more recent. With the transition of yam paracultivators to yam cultivators in the rainforests, human communities established lengthier periods of residency and provided the critical requirement of more continual host density. This created village zones of falciparum infection that exacted high mortality and morbidity costs from hunters and gatherers who could not acquire the limited immunities that came with village life. With the expansion of the zones of yam cultivation, this immunological gradient played a role in the expansion of Bantu-speaking peoples. After the adoption of the plantain / banana complex, rainforest village communities became larger and more stable epidemiologically, and it is in these contexts that the sickle cell mutation spread and that Duffy negativity came closer to its contemporary near universal distribution.

Notes

[1] Reprinted, with permission, from the *Journal of World History* 16 (2005): 269-91. Versions of this essay were presented at the African Studies Seminar at Harvard University; the Science, Technology, and Society Colloquium at Colby College; the African Studies Seminar at Boston University; the History of Economic Development and Growth (HEDG) annual workshop at the School of Oriental and African Studies at the University of London; the biannual meetings of the Society for Africanist Archaeology in Bergen, Norway; and the Health and Medicine in Africa Workshop at Bryn Mawr and Haverford Colleges. I would like to thank Emmanuel Akyeampong, Gareth Austin, Myron Echenberg, Christopher Ehret, H. A. Gemery, Shomarka Keita, Stacey Lance, Scott MacEachern, James McCann, Katharina Neumann, Merrick Posnansky, and Alison Jones Webb for their helpful comments and bibliographic suggestions. A note on the use of time conventions: Archaeologists and microbiologists dealing with periods earlier than ten thousand years ago typically use the convention B.P. (before the present). Scholars working in more recent periods typically use B.C.E. and C.E. In this article, I have used B.P. for periods beginning earlier than ten thousand years ago and B.C.E. for more recent periods. I have chosen to use both conventions in order to avoid the appearance of false precision (e.g., converting 100,000 to 50,000 B.P. to 98,000 to 48,000 B.C.E.).

[2] For a recent effort to bring the early epochs into world history, see David Christians fine introductory chapters "Beginnings: The Era of Foragers" and "Acceleration: The Agrarian Era" in the five-volume *Berkshire Encyclopedia of World History*, ed. William H. McNeill (Great Barrington, Mass.: Berkshire Publishing Group, 2005), 1:1-35.

[3] William H. McNeill, *Plagues and Peoples* (New York: Anchor Books, 1977). McNeill's broad schema has been widely accepted. In a recent authoritative article, David E. Stannard cites McNeill repeatedly in portraying the broad outlines of human disease history. See Stannard, "Disease, Human Migration, and History," in *The Cambridge World History of Human Disease*, ed. Kenneth F. Kiple (Cambridge: Cambridge University Press, 1993), 35-44.

[4] These themes have been reprised to great success by Jared Diamond in his book *Guns, Germs, and Steel* (New York: W. W. Norton & Company, 1997).

[5] For the Cambridge historian John Iliffe, for example, the core theme in African history has been the struggle of Africans to overcome their environment to achieve positive rates of population growth. John Iliffe, *The Africans: History of a Continent* (Cambridge: Cambridge University Press, 1995). Some historians have found Iliffe's insistence on the primacy of this theme in the history of recent centuries to be excessive.

[6] James L. A. Webb Jr., *Desert Frontier: Ecological and Economic Change along the Western Sahel, 1600-1850* (Madison: University of Wisconsin Press, 1995).

[7] Philip D. Curtin, "'The White Man's Grave': Image and Reality, 1780-1850," *Journal of British Studies* 1 (1961): 94-110, and *Death by Migration* (Cambridge: Cambridge University Press, 1989); Dennis G. Carlson, *African Fever: A Study of British Science, Technology, and Politics in West Africa, 1787-1864* (Canton, Mass.: Watson Publishing International, 1984).

[8] There are two other human malarial parasites: *Plasmodium ovale* and *Plasmodium malariae*. Both are far less lethal than falciparum, and they have received less atten-

tion from researchers. Other malaria-protective genetic mutations have emerged within African populations, such as thalassemias, glucose-6-phosphate dehydrogenase deficiency (also known as G6PD deficiency) and hemoglobin C (a genetic variation that is allelic with that for sickle cell but that does not impose as severe costs for individuals who are homozygous for this variation). These polymorphisms are not as protective as Duffy negativity and the sickle cell mutation discussed in this paper. The historical issues concerning the emergence of these polymorphisms have not received as much scientific attention from the molecular biological community.

[9] R. Carter and K. N. Mendis, "Evolutionary and Historical Aspects of the Burden of Malaria," *Clinical Microbiology Reviews* 15 (2002): 564-594.

[10] The deep geographical origin of vivax is contested. One view holds that vivax malaria may have been present in the New World prior to European contact in the late fifteenth and early sixteenth centuries. Although most of the evidence suggests that this was not the case, recently scholars have called for biomolecular analysis of existing skeletal remains in the Amazon to reach a definitive conclusion. See Marcia Caldas de Castro and Burton H. Singer, "Was Malaria Present in the Amazon Before European Conquest? Available Evidence and Future Research Agenda," *Journal of Archaeological Science* 32 (2005): 337-340. The two principal views are that vivax originated either in Africa or in Southeast Asia. Because of the large number of variables and the nature of the evidence, there is latitude for diverse interpretation, and it is unlikely that the issue will be definitively settled. For a recent argument that vivax originated in Southeast Asia, see Ananias A. Escalante, Omar E. Cornejo, Denise E. Freeland, Amanda C. Poe, Ester Durrego, William E. Collins, and Altaf A. Lal, "A Monkey's Tale: The Origin of *Plasmodium Vivax* as a Human Malaria Parasite," *Proceedings of the National Academy of Sciences* 102, (2005): 1980-1985. In this view, vivax never was present in Africa; Duffy antigen negativity is either the result of a genetic accommodation to another, unknown agent or a random genetic variation that became fixed. On the African origins of vivax, see Richard Carter in "Speculations on the Origins of *Plasmodium vivax* Malaria," *Trends in Parasitology* 19, (2003): 214-219. For an overview of some of the complications in unraveling the history of vivax, see Stephen M. Rich, "The Unpredictable Past of *Plasmodium vivax* Revealed in Its Genome," *Proceedings of the National Academy of Sciences* 101 (2004): 15, 547-15, 548.

[11] Duffy antigen negativity (FY*0) is one of three forms of mutation on the Duffy antigen receptor. Duffy A (FY*A) and Duffy B (FY*B) confer limited immunity to malaria. Neither FY*A or FY*B occur in tropical Africa. For more on Duffy mutations, see Martha T. Hamblin and Anna Di Rienzo, "Detection of the Signature of Natural Selection in Humans: Evidence from the Duffy Blood Group Locus," *American Journal of Human Genetics* 66 (2000): 1669-1679; Martha T. Hamblin, Emma E. Thompson, and Anna Di Rienzo, "Complex Signatures of Natural Selection at the Duffy Blood Group Locus," *American Journal of Human Genetics* 70 (2002): 369-383. The biological process is termed "complement fixation." It involves the binding of a "complement" (a heat-sensitive, complex system in fresh human and other sera) to an antigen-antibody complex so that the complement is unavailable for subsequent reaction.

[12] The issue of the evolution of virulence is complex and unresolved. For an introduction, see Alison P. Galvani, "Epidemiology Meets Evolutionary Ecology," *Trends in Ecology and Evolution* 18 (2003): 132-139. See also Margaret J. Mackinnon and Andrew

F. Read, "Virulence in Malaria: An Evolutionary Viewpoint," *Philosophical Transactions of the Royal Society of London, Series B, Biological Sciences* 359 (2004): 965-986.

[13] Human populations apparently were greatly reduced in number, perhaps to as few as five thousand females, around approximately 70,000 B.P. This "population bottleneck" coincides with a cataclysmic eruption of the Toba volcano in Sumatra, which produced a series of volcanic winters. See Stanley H. Ambrose, "Late Pleistocene Human Population Bottlenecks, Volcanic Winter, and Differentiation of Modern Humans," *Journal of Human Evolution* 34 (1998): 623-651; Michael R. Rampino and Stanley H. Ambrose, "Volcanic Winter in the Garden of Eden: The Toba Supereruption and the Late Pleistocene Human Population Crash," in *Volcanic Hazards and Disasters in Human Antiquity*, ed. F. W. McCoy and G. Heiken, *Geological Society of America Special Paper 345* (Boulder, Colo.: Geological Society of America, 2000). For critical interpretations of the Toba eruption and a rejoinder, see F. J. Gathorne-Hardy and W. E. H. Harcourt-Smith, "The Super-Eruption of Toba, Did It Cause a Human Bottleneck?" *Journal of Human Evolution* 45 (2003): 227-230, and Stanley H. Ambrose, "Did the Super-Eruption of Toba Cause a Human Population Bottleneck? Reply to Gathorne-Hardy and Harcourt Smith," *Journal of Human Evolution* 45 (2003): 231-237.

[14] M. T. Hamblin and A. Di Rienzo, the authors of a recent genetic analysis, have proposed that a "selective sweep" toward the fixation of Duffy negativity in sub-Saharan populations began between 97,200 and 6,500 years ago. See their "Detection of the Signature of Natural Selection in Humans," 1669-1679.

[15] For a survey of genetic responses to malarial pressure, including sickle cell (discussed later in the present paper), see Carter and Mendis, "Evolutionary and Historical Aspects," 570-573.

[16] Carter and Mendis, "Evolutionary and Historical Aspects," 577-578. The last glacial maxima in tropical Africa have been estimated at between 22,000 and 12,000. See A. S. Brooks and P. T. Robertshaw, "The Glacial Maxima in Tropical Africa: 22,000-12,000 B.P.," in *The World at 18,000 B.P.: Low Latitudes*, Vol. 2, ed. Olga Soffer and Clive Gamble (London: Unwin Hyman, 1990), 121-169.

[17] The thesis that resistance to malaria is tied to the "agricultural revolution" in Africa is broadly accepted. See, for example, Nina L. Etkin, "The Co-Evolution of People, Plants, and Parasites: Biological and Cultural Adaptations to Malaria," *Proceedings of the Nutrition Society* 62 (2003): 311-317; J. C. C. Hume, J. Lyons, and K. P. Day, "Human Migration, Mosquitoes and the Evolution of *Plasmodium falciparum*," *Trends in Parasitology* 19 (2003): 144-149.

[18] This argument was first advanced by F. B. Livingstone in his classic article "Anthropological Implications of Sickle Cell Gene Distribution in West Africa," *American Anthropologist* 60 (1958): 533-562. Recently, M. Coluzzi has written in support of this thesis in "The Clay Feet of the Malaria Giant and Its African Roots: Hypotheses and Influences About the Origin, Spread, and Control of *Plasmodium falciparum*," *Parassitologia* 41 (1999): 277-283.

[19] John E. Yellen, Alison S. Brooks, Els Cornelissen, Michael J. Mehlman, and Kathlyn Stewart, "A Middle Stone Age Worked Bone Industry from Katanda, Upper Semliki Valley, Zaire," *Science* 268 (1995): 553-556. For the interpretive comparison with Europe, see B. Bower, "African Finds Revise Cultural Roots," *Science News* 147 (1995): 260.

[20] Sally McBrearty and Alison S. Brooks, "The Revolution That Wasn't: A New In-

terpretation of the Origin of Modern Human Behavior," *Journal of Human Evolution* 39 (2000): 458.

[21] Ibid., 532.

[22] Populations that have no immediate experience with malaria can be subject to epidemic malaria. Epidemic malaria is also extremely dangerous. By definition, epidemic outbreaks are episodic; there are fewer prospects for genetic accommodation.

[23] Carter and Mendis, "Evolutionary and Historical Aspects," 573.

[24] For an ambitious, brilliant interpretation of the period 9000-1000 B.C.E., see Christopher Ehret, *The Civilizations of Africa: A History to 1800* (Charlottesville: University of Virginia Press, 2002), 59-158.

[25] Some scholars estimate the period at five to seven million years ago for the divergence of modern falciparum malaria. A. A. Escalante and F. J. Ayala, "Phylogeny of the Malarial Genus *Plasmodium*, Derived from rRNA Gene Sequences," *Proceedings of the National Academy of Sciences USA* 91 (1994): 11, 373-11, 377.

[26] Carter and Mendis, "Evolutionary and Historical Aspects," especially pp. 572 and 578. See also Xin-zhuan Su, Jianbing Mu, and Dierdre Joy, "The 'Malaria's Eve' Hypothesis and the Debate Concerning the Origin of the Human Malaria Parasite *Plasmodium falciparum*," *Microbes and Infection* 5 (2003): 891-896; Daniel L. Hartl, "The Origin of Malaria: Mixed Messages from Genetic Diversity," *Nature Reviews Microbiology* 2 (2004): 15-22.

[27] David J. Conway, "Tracing the Dawn of *Plasmodium falciparum* with Mitochondrial Genome Sequences," *Trends in Genetics* 19 (2003): 671-674. See also David J. Conway, Caterina Fanello, Jennifer M. Lloyd, Ban M. A.-S. Al-Joubori, Aftab H. Baloch, Sushela D. Somanath, Cally Roper, Ayoade M. J. Aduola, Bert Mulder, Marinete M. Povoa, Balbir Singh, and Alan W. Thomas, "Origin of *Plasmodium falciparum* Malaria is Traced by Mitochondrial DNA," *Molecular and Biochemical Parasitology* 111 (2000): 163-171.

[28] David J. Conway and Jake Baum issue a cautionary note on the problems of dating the recent emergence of modern falciparum. See their essay "In the Blood – The Remarkable Ancestry of *Plasmodium falciparum*," *Trends in Parasitology* 18 (2002): 351-355.

[29] Hamblin and Di Rienzo, "Detection of the Signature of Natural Selection in Humans," 1677.

[30] Carter and Mendis, "Evolutionary and Historical Aspects," 571.

[31] Frank B. Livingstone, "Malaria and Human Polymorphisms," *Annual Review of Genetics* 5 (1971): 33-64.

[32] For an overview of the ecological history of West Africa, see James L. A. Webb Jr., "Ecology and Culture in West Africa," in *Themes in West Africa's History*, edited by Emmanuel Akyeampong (Athens: Ohio University Press, 2005), 33-51.

[33] J. G. Vaughn and C. A. Geissler, *The New Oxford Book of Food Plants* (Oxford: Oxford University Press, 1999), 24-25.

[34] M. Adebisi Sowunmi, "The Significance of the Oil Palm (*Elaeis guineensis* Jacq.) in the Late Holocene Environments of West and West Central Africa: A Further Consideration," *Vegetation History and Archaeobotany* 8 (1999): 199-210. These conclusions are tentative, and Sowunmi calls for palynological studies of terrestrial cores and more extensive archaeological study to confirm or refute them. For an interpretation that the expansion of the oil palm was due to climate change, see Jean Maley, with the collaboration of Alex Chepstow-Lusty, "*Elaeis guineensis* Jacq. (Oil Palm) Fluctuations in

Central Africa during the Late Holocene: Climate or Human Driving Forces for This Pioneering Species," *Vegetation History and Archaeobotany* 10 (2001): 117-120.

[35]D. G. Coursey, *Yams: An Account of the Nature, Origins, Cultivation, and Utilisation of the Useful Members of the Dioscoreaceae* (London: Longmans, 1967); D. G. Coursey, "The Origins and Domestication of Yams in Africa," in *Origins of African Plant Domestication*, ed. J. R. Harlan, J. M. J. de Wet, and A. B. L. Stemler (Hague: Mouton, 1975), 383-408.

[36]Edmond Dounias, "The Management of Wild Yam Tubers by the Baka Pygmies in Southern Cameroon," *African Study Monographs*, supp. 26 (2001): 135-156. Dounias defines the term "paracultivation" as "a combination of technical patterns and social rules which structure the exploitation of wild plants. This term characterizes a particular process of wild plant harvesting which aims at encouraging plant reproduction, so that the plant can be repeatedly exploited. Furthermore, the plant is voluntarily kept within its original environment, in order to better respond to the seasonal mobility of forest dwellers. The maintenance of plants in the forest is the key difference between paracultivation and protocultivation" (p. 137).

[37]Christopher Ehret, "Historical/Linguistic Evidence for Early African Food Production," in *From Hunters to Farmers*, ed. J. D. Clark and S. A. Brandt (Berkeley: University of California Press, 1984), 26-39; Ehret, *Civilizations of Africa*, 82-83. The Middle Niger Valley is an important agricultural region in which some dryland crops (notably pennisetum) and the wet crop "red rice" (*Orzya glabberima*) were domesticated. For an excellent overview, see Roderick McIntosh, *The Peoples of the Middle Niger* (Malden, Mass.: Blackwell Publishing, 1998).

[38]Although it is not possible to specify exactly when the sickle cell mutation first developed or became common, specialists are generally agreed that the falciparum malarial parasites developed from within the tropical African woodland and rainforest environments and later spread into other biomes. The earliest human physical evidence of sickle cell anemia comes from the mummified remains of Egyptians from the fourth millennium B.C.E. (A. Marin, N. Cerutti, and E. Rabino Massa, "Use of the Amplification Refractory Mutation System [ARMS] in the Study of HBS in Predynastic Egyptian Remains," *Bollettino della Società Italiana di Biologia Sperimentale* 75 [1999]: 27-30.) This evidence suggests that falciparum may have spread from the upper Nile region to the lower Nile region. The issue of whether or not the sickle cell mutation arose separately in the lower Nile valley remains an open question. Today, the incidence of sickle cell along the entire length of the Nile is very low (0.0-2.5 percent). Stuart Edelstein, *The Sickled Cell: From Myths to Molecules* (Cambridge, Mass.: Harvard University Press, 1986), 148, fig. 7.3.

[39]See, for example, M. E. Kropp Dakubu, "The Peopling of Southern Ghana: A Linguistic Viewpoint," in *The Archaeological and Linguistic Reconstruction of African History*, ed. Christopher Ehret and Merrick Posnansky (Berkeley: University of California Press, 1982), 245-255; and M. E. Kropp Dakubu, "Linguistics and History in West Africa," in Akyeampong, *Themes in West Africa's History*, 52-72.

[40]On the expansion of yam farming in early West Africa, see Bassey W. Andah, "Identifying Early Farming Traditions of West Africa," in *The Archaeology of Africa: Food, Metals and Towns*, ed. Thurston Shaw, Paul Sinclair, Bassey Andah, and Alex Okpoko (New York: Routledge, 1995), 240-254. The expansion of rice farming into the western regions of the West African rainforests is thought to have taken place in the first

millennium C.E.

[41] Kairn Klieman, *"The Pygmies Were Our Compass": Bantu and Batwa in the History of West Central Africa, Early Times to c. 1900 C.E.* (Portsmouth, N.H.: Heinemann, 2003).

[42] E. De Langhe, R. Swennen, and D. Vuylsteke, "Plantain in the Early Bantu World," *Azania* 29-30 (1996): 318-323; Christophe Mindzie Mbida, "Evidence for Banana Cultivation and Animal Husbandry during the First Millennium B.C. in the Forest of Southern Cameroon," *Journal of Archaeological Science* 27 (2000): 151-162; Christophe Mindzie Mbida, "First Archaeological Evidence of Banana Cultivation in Central Africa During the Third Millennium Before Present," *Vegetation History and Archaeobotany* 10 (2001): 1-6.

[43] De Langhe, Swennen, and Vuylsteke, "Plantain," 158, citing Jan Vansina, *Paths in the Rainforests* (Madison: University of Wisconsin Press, 1999).

[44] As Klieman notes, "Bantu populations grew in number, settled into larger more sedentary villages, and began to produce larger quantities and more diverse styles of ceramics. Iron tools and banana cultivation also allowed Bantu villagers to move into forested regions away from the original riverine routes of settlement. This phenomenon resulted in the formation of numerous new speech communities, especially during the Late Stone to Metal Age (1500-500 B.C.E.). As was the case in other parts of Africa, the introduction of iron engendered a greater centralization of local economies and an increase in economic specialization" ('Klieman, *Pygmies Were Our Compass*, 123-124).

[45] Jan Vansina, "New Linguistic Evidence and the 'Bantu Expansion,'" *Journal of African History* 36 (1995): 173-195; Christopher Ehret, "Bantu Expansions: Re-Envisioning a Central Problem of Early African History," *International Journal of African Historical Studies* 34 (2001): 5-41; Roland Oliver, Thomas Spear, Kairn Klieman, Jan Vansina, Scott MacEachern, David Schoenbrun, James Denbow, Yvonne Bastin, H. M. Batibo, and Bernd Heine in "Comments on Christopher Ehret, 'Bantu-History: Re-Envisioning the Evidence of Language,'" *International Journal of African Historical Studies* 34 (2001): 43-87.

[46] Jared Diamond has recently repopularized this notion of a Bantu military-industrial complex (*Guns, Germs, and Steel*, 394-396).

[47] McNeill, *Plagues and Peoples*, 69-131.

[48] This third mutation was first identified in Senegal. Individuals with the Senegalese pattern of sickle cell anemia produce higher levels of hemoglobin F, and this anemia may therefore be less severe. See Edelstein, *Sickled Cell*, 148-149. Experts are not agreed on whether or not sickle cell hemoglobin mutations have a common ancestor. For the argument for a Middle Eastern origin of hemoglobin S and the diffusion of a single mutant, see F. B. Livingstone, "Who Gave Whom Hemoglobin S: The Use of Restriction Site Haplotype Variation for the Interpretation of the Evolution of the β^S-Globin Gene," *American Journal of Human Biology* 1 (1989): 289-302.

[49] Edelstein, *Sickled Cell*, 55-56, 147-148. In the 1980s, it was thought that the two Bantu expansions had taken place in the second and first millennia B.C.E., respectively.

[50] For the argument that population pressure played a major role in prehistory, see Mark Nathan Cohen, *The Food Crisis in Prehistory: Overpopulation and the Origins of Agriculture* (New Haven, Conn.: Yale University Press, 1977).

CHAPTER 9

Drug Resistant Bacteria and Childhood Diarrhea in Africa

FAITH WALLACE-GADSDEN AND IRUKA OKEKE

Every year, 10 million children under the age of five die. Over six million of these children die of preventable causes including acute respiratory infections, diseases for which there are vaccines, and diarrhea.[1] About 90% of these deaths occur in only 42 countries, including 24 sub-Saharan African nations.[2] According to the United Nations Children's Fund (UNICEF), 41% of all childhood deaths occur in this region,[3] and a recent report suggests that 900,000, of these deaths can be attributed to diarrhea.[4] For the children who do not die from these infections, diarrheal disease has important consequences, as it affects growth, development and susceptibility to other infectious diseases. For these reasons, although diarrheal deaths are declining, the adverse impact of the disease continues to exert a very high burden.[5] In this paper, we highlight the continuing threat from infantile diarrhea and the layering of new challenges for controlling the disease. In particular, we focus on enteroaggregative *Escherichia coli*, a pathogen which has been reported from several parts of Africa and is capable of causing persistent diarrhea, but for which routine testing methods do not exist. Although administration of antimicrobial drugs is not advocated for acute diarrhea, antimicrobials can help to prevent growth impairment or death in persistent diarrhea caused by bacteria such as enteroaggregative *E. coli*. Enteroaggregative *E. coli* are frequently drug resistant, a factor that further complicates patient care.

Diarrhea is typically characterized by three or more episodes of semisolid stool a day.[6] It occurs when colonic inflammation inhibits the absorption of liquefied nutrients prior to the stool leaving the body. Because this absorption is inhibited, a large amount of fluids are flushed out of the system, leading to a rapid depletion of water, sodium and nutrients. Children under five years of age may suffer as many as 2.6 incidents of diarrhea a year. In tropical areas, these rates are much higher; studies conducted in parts of India and Brazil report up to 19 episodes a year.[7] Multiple diarrheal incidents are particularly dangerous situations for malnourished children, particularly if they last for more than a few days. Stored nutrients available to 'tide them over' are limited, they will more quickly succumb to dehydration and more severe malnutrition, and are therefore more likely to die or experience repeated episodes. Guerrant et al calculate that repeated bouts diarrhea before age two can be responsible for growth shortfalls of over eight centimeters by age seven, cognitive impairment equivalent to 10 intelligence quotient points, and about one year of schooling, as well as work productivity decreases of as much as 17% due to fitness impairment.[8]

Of the 106.39 million children under the age of five in sub-Saharan Africa, a likely underestimate from the UNICEF,[9] 29% are classified as moderately or severely underweight.[10] Studies have shown that 61% of the children who died from diarrhea in 2000 had malnutrition as an underlying cause of death.[11] These figures illustrate the importance of the cycle of diarrhea and malnutrition. Diarrhea causes malnutrition by preventing the absorption of nutrients, while malnutrition predisposes children to repeated incidents of diarrhea by compromising the immune system, greatly increasing the risk of death from diarrhea. In addition, insufficient hydration and nutrition also leads to stunting, wasting, and what is generally referred to as anthropometric failure.[12]

While diarrhea-associated mortality is falling, morbidity has increased, indicating that Oral Rehydration Therapy has prevented many deaths but the rate of infection has not slowed.[13] According to the UNICEF, only 57% of the population in sub-Saharan Africa has access to water that is likely to be safe. Safe water sources, referred to as "improved drinking water" by the UNICEF and the WHO,[14] include household water connections, public standpipes, boreholes, protected dug wells or springs, and rainwater collection.[15] These sources have a reduced risk of transmitting agents of diarrheal disease. The rest of the population only has access to water that has a greater likelihood of carrying pathogens. In some parts of the continent, the proportion of people exposed to unsafe drinking water is much higher. Additionally, when water is scarce or is difficult and expensive to procure, hand washing is infrequent and person-to-person transfer of infectious material becomes more likely. Improved sanitation systems, including public sewers, connections to a septic system, pour-flush latrines and simple pit latrines are only available to 36% sub-Saharan Africans. Without these basic facilities, communities rely on public latrines, open pit latrines, fields or streams.[16] This improper disposal of waste can lead to the return of pathogens to a community's water and food supply, closing a fecal-oral cycle of infection. The UNICEF and the WHO emphasize breaking this fecal-oral cycle by encouraging covered latrines fully isolated from both the water supply and factors that can return fecal matter to the community. A comparative study conducted in 2005 illustrated the importance of clean drinking water and sanitation. Either improvement can result in a marked reduction in infantile diarrhea.[17] Interventions in hygiene practices, hand washing, and education had a much less significant effect.[18]

While diarrhea prevention has seen little progress, treatment has greatly improved by the inception and application of home-based Oral Rehydration Therapy (ORT). ORT coverage has improved significantly and consequently mortality from diarrheal diseases, although still significant and excessive, has declined over the last three decades. Unfortunately although the WHO recommends that ORT be administered as soon as possible after diarrhea commences, only an estimated 67% of children with diarrhea receive ORT as in accordance with this recommendation.[19] It is therefore critical that health workers and caregivers, who are generally trained through health-worker led educational programs, are fully competent in the preparation and administration of oral rehydration fluids. However, some data suggest that, as much as 90% of all health workers providing pediatric health care are not adequately trained.[20] Studies have shown that in very poor countries, the average child under five has one contact per year with formal allopathic healthcare,[21] mainly at first-level facilities or outpatient clinics, most of which to do not have the resources necessary to manage severely ill children. When the onset of rehydration is delayed, parental rehydration may be the only way to prevent death due to dehydration. For children with limited access to health facilities, referral to a hospital for this more specialized treatment is often logistically difficult or altogether impossible mainly because of cost, distance and difficulty of access.[22]

In an attempt to improve access to optimal care, the WHO and UNICEF have focused attention on the treatment of diarrhea and other common childhood infections by clinic-based healthcare workers through the Integrated Management of Childhood Illness (IMCI). IMCI's core objective is improve childhood survival through training heathcare workers and improving healthcare practices.[23] IMCI recognizes that first-level facilities can potentially identify and treat children who have minor illnesses and require symptomatic or specific treatments. According to WHO recommendations, most cases of diarrhea can be treated in these settings by 1) preventing dehydration, 2) treating dehydration, 3) zinc supplementing, and 4) feeding.[24] In a study conducted in Tanzania, Uganda and Brazil, children treated by an IMCI-trained practitioner were less likely to receive antimicrobials for uncomplicated diarrhea, and other conditions where these drugs are not indicated, than those treated by untrained workers.[25] IMCI workers emphasize the WHO recommendation to replace vital fluids and nutrients to allow the body's immune system clear the infection, and they strongly discourage the use of antibiotics, adsorbents and antimotility drugs. These drugs are not indicated for most cases of diarrhea, can in fact exacerbate the disease, and its overuse promotes the development of resistant bacteria. In cases of suspected cholera or Shigella dysentery, antimicrobials are to be used selectively. Antimicrobials must also be used to address persistent or chronic infections that last more than 14 days.[26] If these recommendations were followed, the WHO estimates that most deaths from acute diarrhea could be eliminated.[27] While the implementation of ORT and continued feeding has improved since the initiative began, the process has been slower in Africa than in other regions.[28]

Although the use of antimicrobial drugs is discouraged by the WHO, in much of Africa its distribution is unregulated. As a result, the public can purchase drugs over-the-counter in pharmacies, general stores and markets without a prescription.[29] Because of the inability for much of the population to access first-level facilities and hospitals, almost half of the children are treated at home.[30] In addition to local methods of managing diarrhea, caretakers often treat children using antibiotics. These drugs are frequently adulterated, "watered down," degraded because of improper storage, or sometimes outright counterfeiting.[31] In addition, improper dispensing and high prices cause them to be bought and sold in quantities too small to clear an infection.[32] When antimicrobials are used in below clinical doses, resistance is more likely to be acquired.

Healthcare providers also inappropriately dispense antimicrobials. Laboratory facilities are not available in most locations, and so often determinations cannot be made as to the best course of treatment in those cases where antimicrobials might be indicated. Patients are usually treated with antimicrobials even when these drugs are not indicated and treatment is inevitably empirical.[33] Public availability combined with inappropriate prescribing leads to the misuse of these agents and the development of resistant bacteria. These resistant strains can then be disseminated in the same ways that other diarrhea-causing bacteria are, via inadequate sanitation, lack of clean water and improper hygiene. The development of resistant bacteria complicates treatment when antimicrobials are indicated, such as in cases of persistent diarrhea or dysentery, and resistant strains can be disseminated locally, regionally, nationally and internationally.

The many micro-organisms that can cause diarrhea include parasites, viruses and bacteria. Health care workers are alert to diarrhea caused by well-known pathogens[34] such as rotavirus, enteric parasites, *Salmonella* species and *Shigella*. With improved detection methods and lifestyle changes, the repertoire of pathogenic organisms continues to grow and change. Diagnostic protocols have not kept pace with these changes so that 'newer' pathogens such as enterohemorrhagic *E. coli*[35] are often undetected. An example pertinent to infantile diarrhea is enteroaggregative *Escherichia coli* (EAEC). This category of *E. coli*, has recently been identified as a major cause of persistent and acute diarrhea worldwide, particularly in Africa.[36] A pathogen of emerging importance that is just beginning to be understood, EAEC is characterized by the "stacked brick" pattern in which it adheres to infected human epithelia cells. This important mechanism contributes to EAEC's ability to cause persistent infections. Children who have persistent or repeated EAEC-mediated diarrhea, as well as children who are infected with EAEC but do not show symptoms, suffer detectable growth impairment.[37]

A number of epidemiological studies in Africa have illustrated a high prevalence of EAEC in both healthy and diarrheal patients. A Kenyan study in 1997 illustrated that persistent diarrhea is associated with drug resistant EAEC.[38] In a 2000 report from Nigeria, EAEC strains were the predominant pathogen found both in diarrheal and healthy children, but were significantly associated with diarrhea.[39] In 2003, a study in Guinea-Bissau showed that EAEC causes 9.7 infections a year, more than any other organism type,[40] and a study in Gabon found EAEC in 38% of children with diarrhea. Although study size and coverage has been small, the wide geographic distribution of these findings illustrates the importance of enteroaggregative *E. coli* in Africa. Few investigators have undertaken studies of EAEC but the pathogen has always been found when it was sought.

Because of the bacteria's ability to cause persistent infections by evading clearance by the immune system, antimicrobials are often indicated for EAEC-mediated infections. EAEC resistance can determine the success of a course of antimicrobials. Techniques for the identification of EAEC are usually performed at specialist laboratories, and are unavailable, even at the tertiary care level, in sub-Saharan Africa. Infections must therefore be treated empirically. In addition to illustrating the distribution and importance of EAEC in diarrhea, studies have also illustrated that these strains have a rate of multiple resistance (resistance to three or more antimicrobials) much higher than other subtypes of *E. coli*. Multiply-resistant EAEC has been reported in Kenya, Tanzania, Senegal, Guinea-Bissau and Nigeria. EAEC has been shown to be resistant to trimethoprim, ampicillin, and tetracycline with prevalence in excess of 50%.[41] In the 2000 Nigerian study, 95.4% of EAEC isolates were tetracycline resistant, 80.9% were ampicillin resistant, and 46.5% were chloramphenicol resistant.[42] Very little work has been done to elucidate resistance mechanisms or describe resistance genes in these organisms. As a result the reason why EAEC has resistance rates that are higher than other *E. coli* remains unclear. Such studies should be prioritized, as should the development of practicable, field diagnostic tests. Although the prominent role that EAEC plays in acute and persistent diarrhea and malnutrition has been highlighted by a number of studies, the question as to how children persistently infected with EAEC should be managed remains to be addressed.[43]

The wide geographic distribution of EAEC, its high rate of antimicrobial resistance, and its ability to mediate persistent infections all come together to make it a very dangerous pathogen. While more research is necessary to elucidate the molecular basis of the high rate of multiple resistance among this population, it is clear that the ongoing misuse of antimicrobials will continue to select for this type of bacteria, and put the children of sub-Saharan Africa at an even greater risk of diarrheal disease. To prevent the spread of and consequences from EAEC infection, it is vital that existing recommendations continue to be implemented. In addition, more attention must be focused on containing the spread of resistance in pathogenic bacteria.

Notes

[1] J. Bryce, S. el Arifeen, G. Pariyo, C. Lanata, D. Gwatkin, and J. P. Habicht, "Multi-Country Evaluation of IMCI Study Group. Reducing Child Mortality: Can Public Health Deliver?" *Lancet* 362 (2003):159-64.

[2] R. E. Black, S. S. Morris, and J. Bryce, "Where and Why Are 10 Million Children Dying Every Year?" *Lancet* 361 (2003): 2226-34.

[3] UNICEF Statistics, "Under Five Mortality Rate" (May, 2004). Available at `http://www.childinfo.org/cmr/revis/db2.htm`.

[4] Black et al, "Where and Why Are 10 Million Children Dying Every Year?"

[5] R. L. Guerrant, R. Oria, O. Y. Bushen, P. D. Patrick, E. Houpt, and A. A. Lima, "Global Impact of Diarrheal Diseases that are Sampled by Travelers: The Rest of the Hippopotamus," *Clinical Infectious Diseases*, 41 (2005), Suppl.: S524-30.

[6] WHO, "Diarrhoea Treatment Guidelines January, 2005," `http://www.who.int/child-adolescent-health/New_Publications/CHILD_HEALTH/Diarrhoea_guidelines.pdf`.

[7] S. R. Moore, A. A. Lima, M. R. Conaway, J. B. Schorling, A. M. Soares, and R. L. Guerrant, "Early Childhood Diarrhoea and Helminthiases Associated with Long-Term Linear Growth Faltering, *International Journal of Epidemiology* 30 (2001): 1457-64.

[8] Guerrant et al, "Global Impact of Diarrheal Diseases."

[9] UNICEF Global Database on Child Malnutrition, `http://www.childinfo.org/eddb/malnutrition/database1.htm`.

[10] UNICEF Monitoring and Statistics, `http://www.unicef.org/statistics/`.

[11] Black et al, "Where and Why Are 10 Million Children Dying Every Year?"

[12] S. Nandy, M. Irving, D. Gordon, S. V. Subramanian, and G. D. Smith, "Poverty, Child Undernutrition and Morbidity: New Evidence from India." *Bulletin of the World Health Organization* 83 (2005): 210-6.

[13] Guerrant et al, "Global Impact of Diarrheal Diseases."

[14] WHO, "2004 Definitions of Indicators: Meeting the MDG Drinking Water and Sanitation Target," `http://www.unicef.org/wes/mdgreport/definition.php`.

[15] WHO, "Definitions of Indicators."

[16] WHO, "Definitions of Indicators."

[17] L. Fewtrell, R. B. Kaufmann, D. Kay, W. Enanoria, L. Haller, and J. M. Colford, Jr., "Water, Sanitation, and Hygiene Interventions to Reduce Diarrhoea in Less Developed Countries: A Systematic Review and Meta-Analysis." *Infectious Diseases* 5 (2005): 42-52.

[18] Fewtrell et al, "Water, Sanitation, and Hygiene Interventions."

[19] UNICEF Monitoring and Statistics, `http://www.unicef.org/view_chart.php?sid=2ef6b9ce415e2815c2293a673f15f946&create_chart=Create+Table+%3E%3E&submit_to_chart=1&layout=1&language=eng`.

[20] Bryce et al, "Multi-Country Evaluation of IMCI Study Group."

[21] Bryce et al, "Multi-Country Evaluation of IMCI Study Group."

[22] E. A. Simoes, S. Peterson, Y. Gamatie, F. S. Kisanga, G. Mukasa, J. Nsungwa-Sabiiti, and M.W. Weber, "Management of Severely Ill Children at First-Level Health Facilities in Sub-Saharan Africa when Referral is Difficult," *Bulletin of the World Health Organization* 81 (2003): 522-31.

[23] S. Gove, "Integrated Management of Childhood Illness by Out Patient Heath Work-

ers: Technical Basis and Overview," *Bulletin of the World Health Organization* 75, Suppl 1 (1997): 25-32.

[24]WHO Diarrhoea Treatment Guidelines.

[25]E. Gouws, J. Bryce, J. P. Habicht, J. Amaral, G. Pariyo, J. A. Schellenberg, and O. Fontaine, "Improving Antimicrobial Use Among Health Workers in First-Level Facilities: Results From the Multi-Country Evaluation of the Integrated Management of Childhood Illness Strategy." *Bulletin of the World Health Organization* 82(2004): 509-15.

[26]P. K. Muhuri, M. Anker, and J. Bryce, "Treatment Patterns for Childhood Diarrhoea: Evidence from Demographic and Health Surveys," *Bulletin of the World Health Organization* 74 (1996): 135-46.

[27]WHO Diarrhoea Treatment Guidelines.

[28]See http://www.unicef.org/mdg/index.html.

[29]I. N. Okeke, A. Lamikanra, and R. Edelman, "Socioeconomic and Behavioral Factors Leading to Acquired Bacterial Resistance to Antibiotics in Developing Countries," *Emerging Infectious Diseases* 5 (1999): 18-27.

[30]Muhuri et al, "Treatment Patterns for Childhood Diarrhoea."

[31]Okeke et al, "Socioeconomic and Behavioral Factors."

[32]C. M. Kunin, "Use of Antimicrobial Drugs in Developing Countries," *International Journal of Antimicrobial Agents* 5 (1995): 107-113.

[33]C. A. Hart, and S. Kariuki, "Antimicrobial Resistance in Developing Countries," *British Medical Journal* 317 (1998): 647-50.

[34]A pathogen is a micro-organism that causes disease.

[35]Enterohemorrhagic *E. coli*, typified by *E. coli* O157, is known to be an important diarrheal pathogen in Europe, North America and Japan. It was previously thought not to be prevalent in Africa, but recent etiologic studies have shown that this idea is a misconception.

[36]W. K. Sang, J. O. Oundo, J. K. Mwituria, P. G. Waiyaki, M. Yoh, T. Iida, and T. Honda, "Multidrug-Resistant Enteroaggregative *Escherichia coli* Associated with Persistent Diarrhea in Kenyan Children," *Emerging Infectious Diseases* 3 (1997): 373-4; I. C. A. Scaletsky, M. L. M. Silva, and L. R. Trabulsi, "Distinctive Patterns of Adherence of Enteropathogenic *Escherichia coli* to Hela Cells," *Infection and Immunity* 45 (1984): 534-6; I. N. Okeke, I. C. Scaletsky, E. H. Soares, L. R. Macfarlane, and A. G. Torres, "Molecular Epidemiology of the Iron Utilization Genes of Enteroaggregative *Escherichia coli*," *Journal of Clinical Microbiology* 42 (2004): 36-44.

[37]T. S. Steiner, A. A. Lima, J. P. Nataro, and R. L. Guerrant, "Enteroaggregative *Escherichia coli* Produce Intestinal Inflammation and Growth Impairment and Cause Interleukin-8 Release from Intestinal Epithelial Cells," *Journal of Infectious Diseases* 177 (1998): 88-96.

[38]Sang et al, "Multidrug-Resistant Enteroaggregative *Escherichia coli*."

[39]I. N. Okeke, A. Lamikanra, J. Czeczulin, F. Dubovsky, J. B. Kaper, and J. P. Nataro, "Heterogeneous Virulence of Enteroaggregative *Escherichia coli* Strains Isolated from Children in Southwest Nigeria." *Journal of Infectious Diseases* 181 (2000): 252-60.

[40]H. Steinsland, P. Valentiner-Branth, M. Perch, F. Dias, T. K. Fischer, P. Aaby, K. Molbak, and H. Sommerfelt, "Enterotoxigenic *Escherichia coli* Infections and Diarrhea in a Cohort of Young Children in Guinea-Bissau," *Journal of Infectious Diseases* 186 (2002): 1740-7.

[41] Okeke at al, "Heterogeneous Virulence of Enteroaggregative *Escherichia coli* Strains."

[42] Okeke at al, "Heterogeneous Virulence of Enteroaggregative *Escherichia coli* Strains."

[43] R. L. Guerrant, T. Van Gilder, T. S. Steiner, N. M. Thielman, L. Slutsker, R. V. Tauxe, T. Hennessy, P. M. Griffin, H. DuPont, R. B. Sack , P. Tarr, M. Neill, I. Nachamkin, L. B. Reller, M. T. Osterholm, M. L. Bennish, and L. K. Pickering, "Infectious Diseases Society of America: Practice Guidelines for the Management of Infectious Diarrhea," *Clinical Infectious Diseases* 32 (2001): 331-51.

CHAPTER 10

Classify and Sequestrate: The Regulation of Madness in Saint-Louis du Sénégal, 1890-1914

KALALA NGALAMULUME

In 1892 Jules B., a colonial administrator in Saint-Louis, capital of French Senegal, aged thirty-eight years, experienced a mental breakdown. On several occasions, his neighbor, Ballacey, reported being the subject of verbal abuse and threats, as well as witnessing instances of domestic violence against Jules' wife, to whom he provided assistance. One of his letters to the Prosecutor of the Republic was very explicit. "I have alerted the city's Sergeant several times," he wrote in 1892. After describing the problems he was having with Jules, he concluded:

> You understand, Mr. Prosecutor, that it is not reassuring to have a neighbor who is becoming more and more insane. If he starts with threats, he will end up shooting at us, for not long ago he bought a rifle and a handgun in the city and from a man who is out of his mind, one can fear anything. I have warned Mr. Aumont who is the owner of the building where my neighbor lives.[1]

But it took five years, until December 1897, for the authorities to arrest Jules B. and to incarcerate him in the Military Hospital. By then, he had become increasingly "dangerous for the public security."[2] The list of his transgressions had become very long, including violence against the couple Ndiaye, threats to neighbors, and monomania (or "mania of persecution").[3] Even then, the Prosecutor of the Republic who requested his arrest did so reluctantly. The confinement of Jules B. sent a wave of consternation among the administration officials and his relatives in France. In the context characterized by colonial mythologies about racial susceptibility and about the inability of Africans to cope with colonial modernity,

Jules B.'s case became a real embarrassment for the white community. After forty-three days of clinical observation, the *Médecin en Chef* saw little improvement in his condition and, on March 25, 1898, he transferred him to the Marseille Public Lunatic Asylum in accordance with the existing treaty.[4] Jules' name continued to appear on the yearly general registry of the asylum but, after 1905, he disappeared from the records.[5] Jules B. was not the only white insane in Saint-Louis. There were two others, Barrère and Rebours. But unlike Jules B., they did not leave behind their own stories.

Jules B.'s case is interesting in that it sheds light on the presuppositions of early colonial psychiatry and the knowledge it generated, the intentions of the French health authorities, the experience of the sufferer from the sufferer's point of view, and, through his delusions, his anxieties and preoccupations, as well as those of the colonial society. His story and other cases of insanity observed in Saint-Louis from the 1890s onwards also help us understand the ways in which relatives of the insane interacted with colonial health institutions. Dealing with the insane posed new challenges to the health officers who were so far preoccupied with the most visible pathologies of colonialism in a colony not equipped with lunatic asylums and health professionals.

Previous studies on the history of psychiatry, mental illness, and asylums in colonial Africa have provided useful insights into the dynamics of the colonial state; the political and cultural conflict between Africans and Europeans;[6] the colonial mentality and the limits of colonial psychiatry in understanding, with its clinical vocabulary, the psychology of Africans;[7] and the perspectives of the patients.[8] The existing literature has also shown that Michel Foucault's claim about the insane "great confinement" is not supported by the evidence from African colonial situations, given the low rank that madness occupied on the list of health priorities of colonial officials, the small number of black insane who were institutionalized, the lack of funds and personnel,[9] and the inclusion of the 'lepers' and the 'chronic sick' among the 'lunatics.'[10] Foucault's use of highly selective French material to represent the entire Western world has also recently come under attack from British sociologist Andrew Shull.[11]

Despite this clear lack of interest in mental illness on the part of colonial authorities compared to the more threatening epidemic and endemic diseases, colonial psychiatry did play an important role, not only in accentuating social control but also, and more importantly, in providing additional racialized knowledge that, as pointed out by James H. Mills concerning British India, had "the power to construct standards of normality and deviancy and of morality and immorality,"[12] and was used for the construction of "the African" as "the Other," as "primitive" and "savage."[13] In addition, these studies have emphasized the fact that far from being fully controlled by physicians and the state, the asylum itself was "a contested site, subject to continual negotiation amongst different parties, including families and the patients themselves."[14] Social historians of medicine in colonial contexts have pointed to the importance of constantly questioning the diagnosis of the inmates of the asylums as insane, and of analyzing the statements and actions of those incarcerated.[15]

Psychiatric therapeutics and practice in Sénégal were given momentum by the Dakar school of African ethnopsychiatry, founded in 1958 by Professor H. Collomb and his collaborators, who sought to break away from the colonial model and to understand and treat madness in its wider social and cultural context of post-independence Senegal. The Dakar school has provided material for the understanding of the history of psychiatry in Senegal in the past three decades, as illustrated in the articles published in the *Psychopathologie africaine*; but there are few published historical studies on madness and colonialism in Senegal. Historians Mamadou Diouf and Mohammed Mbodj have, in a 1997 book chapter, provided an administrative history of madness in Senegal in which they presented a general overview of the attempts made by French colonial authorities to deal with madness in Senegal between 1840 and 1956.[16] But more scholarship is needed to deal with the experience of the sufferers. This study tries to fill the gap by shedding light on the confinement system, the agency of the family and relatives, and the patients' perspective, using previously unexamined archival materials.

Responding to the deranged: the confinement system

The available historical evidence suggests that before the 1890s French colonial officials did not consider insanity among those classified as *indigènes* as requiring an institutional response. The native mad were kept at home or left to roam the city streets and Saint-Louis' hinterland. Although ordinances were issued to regulate the movement of the floating population in the city, comprising vagabonds, beggars, prostitutes, and people without fixed domicile, no particular attention was given to the native deranged. But in 1890 things changed, and the records indicate that twenty native insane were incarcerated in the Civilian Hospital.[17] Insanity became a medical problem probably because of the growth of the urban population, which pressured the colonial administration officials to try to model the city residents' social behavior around the norms of rational bourgeois expectations. Even then, the decision to round up the "mad" people, and sequestrate them in the hospital or in the prison, was made with the full knowledge that there were no "mad doctors" in Saint-Louis, so the existing physicians had to extend their claims to new areas of medical practice and to deploy the unfamiliar lexicon of madness, insanity, and lunacy.

After 1890, socially problematic and disruptive individuals were considered *aliéné(e)*[18] or insane. However, there was no asylum in Saint-Louis, and the law of June 30, 1838 that had provisions for the *placement d'office*, or official committal, of "the patient (who) is a danger to him/herself or to others," was not implemented. Instead, the governor made use of an ordinance of September 7, 1840 related to the maintenance of law and order, to deal with the disturbances caused by the lunatics.[19] Some insane were apprehended by the police and taken to the Civilian Hospital – or to the Military Hospital in the case of European soldiers and civil servants – on the recommendation of the police chief. Other insane who posed serious threats to the families or local community were also sent to the hospital. The majority of the insane was incarcerated after disturbing law and order so as to prevent further "unconscious infractions they can commit anytime."[20] Likewise, neighbors could denounce individuals who posed threats to the community. Convicts and the indigents were also among the insane. So the *aliéné* category encompassed a variety of conditions, ranging from idiocy, to dementia and melancholia, and all types of mania (monomania, mania of persecution, and furious mania, to name the most commonly used). At the hospital, the patient was examined by the *Médecin des Affaires Indigènes* after a period of observation; then the physician established a diagnosis and recommended hospitalization.

The available case files show that mental patients were classified according to how refractory they were. There were two categories of lunatics, the non-criminal lunatics and the dangerous or criminal lunatics. The non-criminal lunatics, with less disruptive forms of insanity, were the mentally ill who did not disturb public order, but who became a burden for their families and needed treatment they could not provide. Among these, doctors considered those harmless mental patients unable to live a normal and independent life because of either mental deficiencies (such as imbecility) or neurological disorders (such as epilepsy). Criminal lunatics were classified according to different categories of mania. They were taken into custody by the police after exhibiting disruptive conduct, and transferred to the Civilian Hospital, where they were classified according to their behavior. Between 1890 and 1910, the main categories of "dangerous insanity" comprised several types of mania that can be translated into modern psychiatric language as schizophrenia, manic depression, obsessive-compulsory disorder, and suicidal depression. But in the 1890s the psychiatric categories were vague and ambiguous.

Those who were labeled insane were subjugated to a strict surveillance, to which many patients opposed a determined resistance. In a confidential letter to the Interior Director, after two months of sequestration in the Military Hospital in Saint-Louis, Jules provided unique insights into the custodian system. He complained that for fifty-seven days he was not allowed to receive visits from his pregnant "legitimate wife" and his daughter; and that he was left "without knowing exactly what [was] going on at home." From his perspective, in the light of his "excellent health" for a "seasoned civil servant in warm climates and destined to serve in the 'bush'", the whole situation looked "abnormal," and he revealed that his sequestration was causing him "considerable moral and material prejudice." He asked the Interior Director to obtain from the Governor General compensation for such treatment.[21] This letter, written by Jules probably during his moments of quietude, underlines the insensitivity of the medical authorities, who did not take into account the specific circumstances of each patient. It is not clear whether the authorities' refusal to allow Jules' family to visit him was motivated by racial prejudice (his wife being black) or by the genuine concern for his mental state and its effects on his family.

The conditions of confinement that transpire from Jules' file are corroborated by evidence from other insane Frenchmen. Barrère, a French citizen whose occupation was not provided, was admitted to the Civilian Hospital for "violent over-excitations." His level of violence prompted the authorities to add metallic bars to the window of his room and a special lock to the door in order to prevent him from escaping. His condition was labeled '*lypémania*.' Rebours, clerk in the Interior Affairs bureau, experienced general paralysis before exhibiting signs of mania of persecution. He was transferred to a "special (medical) facility" in the Var *département* in France.[22] It should be underlined that the description of the symptoms and the psychiatric labels used to classify the insane did not make a clear distinction between different types of insanity, and the line between the sane people and the deranged was a blurry one. The *Médecin en Chef* acknowledged the possibility of misdiagnosis in a correspondence to the Governor General. He confessed that the diagnosis of mental afflictions among the *indigènes* [was] surrounded with such difficulties that several physicians agreed not to give a label before a sufficient period of observation either at the garrison, at the hospital, or the prison.[23] But what appears more clearly is the fact that the labeling process was informed by both racial and gendered conceptions of the body.

The evidence presented here shows that the functions of the police, responsible for maintaining law and order, extended to the realm of medicine. Police defined mental patients as those who acted in a way contrary to public morals, arrested them and sent them to the hospital for incarceration. Here the hospital played the role of a normalizing institution that Michel Foucault attributed to workhouses, schools, prisons, almshouses, and asylums.[24] Given that the two hospitals were not equipped to provide treatment and cure for the insane, their sequestration could only be understood in the framework of maintaining social control over the urban poor – and, in the case of the Europeans, a way of protecting a certain image of the European in the colony. In the absence of an asylum, the authorities saw the custodian system as a temporary solution to the problem of insanity. The *Médecin en Chef* took considerable pain to demonstrate the uselessness of the sequestration policy. Referring to Jules' situation, he argued that

> The [hospital] cell is not a means of treating an insane, but should rather be an extreme resource to put him/her in the impossibility to harm [others] during specific crises of excitation ... we don't have the means not only to cure him, but also to simply care for him. We are only feeding him. Unfortunately, we are also sequestrating him. That is contrary to the most elementary rules of the therapy of mental illnesses, and is certainly harmful to our pensioner. That is, indeed, a new persecution that we add on top of the other [persecutions] that he is already subject to in his imagination.[25]

This process of framing insanity in Senegal sheds light on the emerging racialized and gendered psychiatric knowledge and the problems encountered in its application in a colonial city.

The agency of the family

The intervention of the patient's family underlined the contested nature of colonial medical institutions. Jules' wife does not figure in the official records, but reactions from his relatives in France help us understand the struggle for defining madness. Not only were Jules's relatives attempting to obtain his discharge from the hospital, or at least changes in the terms of his confinement, but they also put forward their own diagnosis of his condition. Indeed, Jules's relatives were the first to try to make sense of this tragedy. According to them, Jules had experienced mental breakdown within two years after he returned from a ten-month mission of inspection and exploration in Congo in 1890, ordered by General Commissar Savorgnan de Brazza.

Camille R., Jules' brother-in-law based in Lyons (France), suggested that during his trip to Congo Jules had suffered from "isolation that almost cost him his life and from which he never recovered"[26] and, at the end of 1895, from "cerebral anemia" for which he received a three-month medical leave that, unfortunately, did not bring him healing. Camille also established a direct link between Jules' mental illness and his unexpected and "strange" marriage in 1896 to a "négresse," a Malinke woman with whom he had a baby named Marie, as well as his bizarre resignation at the end of the year from his important position of colonial administrator. Camille concluded that Jules' "dementia" resulted from the "fatigue accumulated during his trip at the service of the State" and "from the isolation he had experienced while in Congo."[27] How did the medical authorities respond to Camille? Further research is needed to answer this question; but his strict confinement and transfer to Marseille suggest that his request was not granted.

Jules B.'s perspective

Arguing against biological psychiatric theories that dismiss the stories of mental patients as nonsense, scholars such as Ann Braden Johnson and

Jonathan Sadowsky have suggested that the words and bizarre behavior of mental patients contain messages that must be decoded for political and religious meanings.[28]

Jules B. wrote about various issues. At the beginning of his psychological breakdown, Jules strongly protested against his conditions of detention, which he felt were inhumane and frankly arbitrary. Besides voicing his opposition against the confinement system, Jules' first preoccupation was with his personal safety, the welfare of his family, and his career. In April 1897, Jules B. offered a different explanation for his resignation from his important position. Indeed, he accused Police Chief Morau R. for allowing people to insult him, and it was those insults that led him to resign from his position of Colonial Administrator. He affirmed that the insults were also directed against his wife's reputation with the intended goal of pushing her to divorce him and to keep the custody of their child. At stake was his personal reputation and that of his family, especially his father. For this abuse of power and official misconduct of Police Chief, Jules requested a compensation of 100,000 francs.[29]

In June, Jules complained against his neighbor Ballacey for insulting him, bewitching and persecuting both him and his daughter, violating the secret of his correspondence, uttering death threats and rape threats against his wife, and threatening to kidnap his daughter. He wrote that

> Not content to repeatedly insult me in conversations held in the public space, Mr. Ballacey had me materially bewitched by people unknown to me. That bewitchment has extended to my little daughter, aged 20 months. I came to the point where I could not write a Letter, read, or receive a Correspondence, without that being known and commented upon in the neighborhood, even if I did not tell anybody. In these conditions, having received death threats, rape threats against my legitimate wife, and abduction threats against my only child, etc. etc. ...I have the honor to request that you use your high authority in order for me to be respected ... by Mr. Ballacey, as well as different neighbors I do not know and against whom I have already made verbal complaints at the Police Station in Sor as well as at the main Commissariat, at the office of the Prosecutor of the Republic and at the General Parquet.[30]

He expressed fear that his (imaginary or real) enemies would try to cause him harm. Using the witchcraft idiom, he also accused Merlin, probably another colonial official, of bewitching him through intermediaries, and he mentioned specific dates and locations where this took place, such as on the terrace of the *Cercle*, in the dining hall of the hospital, and in Merlin's office. Jules stated that the bewitchment and persecution were aimed at pushing his wife to divorce him. He wrote that he overheard "Ballay tanzi, or protestant Makana" saying that "I intend to push her for divorce as we did for Boundoute." Jules saw the development of a wide conspiracy against him that also involved the Catholic Church. One Sunday evening, as the nuns were returning from the city-island to their Convent in Sor quarter, Jules was "very surprised to see one of them (maybe a novice) looking with obstinacy through the Moorish mats trying to see, me, my wife or my child, and repeating words that I did not understand the content of."[31]

A careful reading of Jules' notes reveals the prevailing negative attitude among the French populace toward the Europeans who married or cohabited with native women. Indeed, Jules' fear was that his enemies would break his marriage. How can we explain the absence of his wife's name in the correspondence not only from Jules himself (understandable, given his circumstances), but also from people around him? His neighbor Ballacey referred to Jules' wife simply as "*une négresse,*" "*sa femme,*" and "*sa négresse.*"[32] In a letter to the Minister of Colonies, Camille mentioned her as a "*Malanke (Malinké?)* woman," thus highlighting her position as an ultimate "Other."[33] It is not at all clear how to interpret such silence; was it an indication of the rise of intolerance toward interracial unions or simply an expression of patriarchal attitudes? More evidence is needed to answer this question. A second set of issues in Jules' delusions have religious and political meanings. Indeed, Jules' statement that "those who have read the book *Diable au XIXème Siècle* must *die* or *confess* the Divinity of Christ" could be interpreted as a reference to the debates over the rise of anticlericalism that characterized the 1880s and 1890s in France and the colonies. In one note, Jules wrote:

> Every night, they ask me if I know anything about infanticide, then about the suicide of Carbucero, – about the secret of Amhadou Bamba – about the Dahomean bewitchers, about the nihilists who have the intention of blowing up the new bridge of Saint-Louis, on the day of its inauguration.[34]

In this piece of evidence transpire the intentions and obsessive dispositions of Jules' enemies who, through repeated interrogations ("every night"), allegedly threatened his life. His persecutors operated at night, precisely when witches were believed to go out in spirit to decide about the fate of their victims, and to engage in mystical feasting. The colonial medical, as well as missionary, discourses frequently used the idiom of witchcraft to make sense of the indigenous conceptions of health and disease and of the resistance of the local population to aspects of Western medicine.

The reference to the kingdom of Dahomey makes sense in the context of ongoing military operations against King Behanzin of Dahomey. Indeed, the French troops led by General Alfred-Amédée won a major victory at Abomey in 1892, the same year when Jules' mental disturbance began. General Dodds, from a leading Creole family, was then praised as the *vainqueur du Dahomey* (the conqueror of Dahomey). The conquest of Abomey was followed by the French declaration of a protectorate over the entire kingdom; King Behanzin was deported to Martinique. But the association of Dahomey with witchcraft in Jules' mind certainly related to the widespread practice of *Vodun* and the prominent role women ("bewitchers") played in the political and religious spheres of the kingdom. Dahomey provided ethnologists and adventurers with the needed "evidence" of superstition and cannibalism that the civilizing mission had to wipe out.

The reference to Ahmadou Bamba, a Muslim cleric founder of the Mourid brotherhood in Senegal, can also be understood in the context of the colonial conquest of Senegal. French authorities had classified Amadou Bamba as an enemy who posed a serious threat to the viability of French rule in Senegal, and they were determined to neutralize him. In August 1895, he was arrested and jailed in Saint-Louis, before being deported first to Gabon in September of the same year, then to Mauritania in June 1903, and finally returning to Senegal in 1907.[35] These current affairs were widely discussed in the colonial circles where Jules occupied an important position. Thus, Jules' delusions reveal some of the preoccupations and anxieties of the colonial authorities: the colonial expansion in West Africa and the resistance to it, the separation between the Church and the State, as well as the agency of local centrifugal forces within the French community (the "nihilists" and others).

How did Jules B. see himself? Although a member of the colonial elite, he would have been perceived in colonial circles as an eccentric fellow because of his psychiatric disturbance that resulted in a marriage to a *négresse*.[36] Nevertheless, he saw himself as a middleman between the colonizers and the colonized. The go-in-between position was an important asset that he was prepared to use when, after four months of treatment in the Marseille asylum, he sent a letter to the Interior Director in Saint-Louis offering his services to the colonial state, preferably in Saint-Louis, where he had left his pregnant wife and their daughter Marie. He explained that "thanks to [his] immediate kinship relations with the black race, [he could] – by taking care in a special manner of the indigenous prisoners, render great services to the Colony."[37]

The Senegalese insane

Unlike Jules, the overwhelming majority of the insane in Saint-Louis were members of the so-called undisciplined urban underclass, and predominantly men. The Director of the Marseille Asylum described the majority of those who were dispatched there as "the patients from Senegal who did not understand nor speak the French language."[38] A few among them held poorly paid jobs, such as domestic servants, laundry workers and service workers; only four could be classified as skilled workers, including one mechanic and three riflemen. The rest were poor individuals being cared for by unemployed or underemployed relatives who were themselves experiencing difficult living conditions. The social background of these patients can help explain the silence of African voices in the official records, besides the voices filtered through the comments of the authorities in their correspondence.

Non-criminal lunatics were chronic, long-stay patients in the hospital. Samba M., incarcerated for eight years on police order, was described as "childlike with weak spirit, but docile, helpful and affectionate to his protectors." He was not considered a danger to society. For this reason, he was given complete freedom "as long as children were not mean to him." Barrick, diagnosed with "ambitious madness" and "melancholia," during his seventh year of confinement was not a danger to those around him. But during his moments of madness, he spoke and referred to himself as "God, governor, and owner of the whole world." These episodes were followed by periods of dumbness and "melancholia." Abel P., aged thirty-five years, was deaf, blind, and dumb but noisy, and uttered inarticulate screams. His life was reduced to eating, drinking, smoking, and sleeping. He was on his seventh year of surveillance at the hospital. Sacco M, a former *tirailleur* (rifleman), was interned for "maniac excitations" that consisted of singing, laughing, and making a racket, but without meanness. His status was that of an "idiot doubled with non dangerous mania."[39]

Criminal lunatics, on the contrary, were mentally ill and harmful patients, who had to remain under constant surveillance for the rest of their lives. Although the admission procedure is not made explicit in these cases, the evidence seems to indicate that the police played an important role in their confinement, even if some of them were admitted on a voluntary basis. Sihr B., a thirty-year-old resident of Bouteville quarter, entered the train station and attacked the crew members. Under interrogation, he responded with "incoherent words." He was sent to the civilian hospital. Anna C. was noisy, quarrelsome, and always ready to bite anyone approaching her. She was under "continuous surveillance" for six years. Yena A., a trader aged thirty-five years, was diagnosed with "mania of persecution," which made her violent. Moumar D. was, on his father's demand, brought to Saint-Louis from his village of Hainoumale (Bakel), where he was engaged in activities characteristic of a "dangerous madman," such as "troubling the security of the whole village." Upon arrival in Saint-Louis, the police took him to the hospital for observation and diagnosis. His fate is unknown.[40] Mamadou A., a *tirailleur* serving two years after his conviction for desertion, was diagnosed with "acute mania, signs of degeneracy; permanent excitation; incoherence of ideas; periods of hallucination, [and] religious mania (occasionally)." His case file indicates that he "engage[d] in daily irrational acts of hearing and vision."[41] In the case of Fatimata T., a fifty-year-old former domestic servant, dangerousness was attributed to her alleged, but not demonstrated, sexual behavior. She was arrested and confined to the hospital because she engaged in "acts contrary to public morality." Her condition was labeled "erotic madness," requiring treatment in a "special hospital" elsewhere. Her case indicates the sexualized nature of disease categorization.

Table 10.1 provides a summary of the profiles of the insane patients for whom records survived. The examination of this table suggests that after 1898 there was a temporary halt on the transfer of the insane to France, for reasons that still need to be elucidated. In 1908, it appears that the seven mental patients listed are the chronically ill who were diagnosed with noncriminal madness. The evidence supporting such assertion is the presence of Sihr B. on that list, the other patients being Kante K., Ndiaye M., Kane B., Pate M., Fatou, and a woman whose name is not provided.

Table 10.1: Profiles of 27 Black Insane Patients, Senegal, 1890s

Name	Age	Sex	Occupation	Diagnosis	Transfer to Marseille	Outcome
Temba L.	-	M	Rifleman	Insane	-	-
Mama S.	-	M	Rifleman	Insane	-	-
Mamadou A.	-	M	Rifleman	Acute mania	-	-
Fatimata T.	50	F	Maid	Erotic madness	-	-
Barrick F.	-	-	-	Insane	7-17-1897	-
Coumba K.D	-	M	-	Insane	7-17-1897	-
Fatimata M.	28	F	Maid	Insane	7-17-1897	Died on 7-13-1898
Ibrahima C.	-	M	-	Insane	7-17-1897	-
Moddy B.	-	-	-	Insane	7-17-1897	-
Sacco M.	-	-	-	Insane	7-17-1897	-
Sadio S.	-	-	-	Insane	7-17-1897	-
Seck C.	28	M	Mechanic	Insane	7-17-1897	Recovered
Tabara D.	-	M	-	Insane	7-17-1897	-
Temba L.	-	M	-	Insane	7-17-1897	-
Yena A.	35	F	Retailer	Insane	7-10-1897	Died en route
Balla N.	-	-	-	Insane	3-15-1898	-
Bambie S.	-	-	-	Insane	3-15-1898	-
Khary G.	40s	-	-	Insane	3-15-1898	-
Marouba T.	20	M	-	Insane	3-15-1898	-
Samba N.	-	-	-	Insane	3-15-1898	-
Moumar D.	-	M	-	Divine madness	No	-
She B.	-	M	-	Mental impairment	No	Released to his family
Dioga B.	29	M	-	Mental impairment	No	-
Sihr B.	30	M	-	Insane	No	-
Abel P.	35	M	-	Mental impairment	No	-
Anna C.	-	F	-	Insane	No	-

TABLE SOURCE: "Assistance publique: Admission des malades mentaux à l'Hospice Civil, 27 janvier – 23 décembre 1896-1898, " ANS/H45/Sénégal.

Elements for the construction of a specific form of racial psychiatry, that is, for the creation of black Muslims as the other, appear in the correspondence concerning Moumar B. and Sihr B., where religious explanations of acute mental illness emphasize the danger associated with the study of Islam. Indeed, during his transfer from one jurisdiction to another, several authorities depicted Moumar as a "fanatic," a "dangerous fanatic," and "an *indigène* who claims to be animated by the divine spirit, a very dangerous madman."[42] This condition, called mystic madness, thought to be "frequent among students of Arabic." Another case in point is Sihr B., who covered the walls of his cell with Koranic prayers and answered questions with prayer formulas. He claimed to be surrounded by spiders and insects. One of his acquaintances, Boubacar, explained that Sihr "had studied too much Arabic and oftentimes that exaltation happens to one of us because of our study, which happens a lot mostly among the Toucouleur marabouts during the period of apprenticeship."[43]

It must be emphasized that in order to get his relative released to the family, Boubacar's request to the authorities had to fit in with the official thinking among law enforcement authorities about what happens to social actors who depart from institutionalized normative patterns; by studying "too much Arabic," the *talibés* (*madrasa* students) broke cultural codes and became deviants, insane. In Boubacar's explanation there is also an attempt to single out an ethnic group, the Toucouleur (or Puular), as mainly responsible for the production of this new social pathology. It is clear that a crisis of faith had no place in the colonial categories; an Islamic puritan was simply labeled a fanatic and a threat to social order in Senegal. Thus the labels applied to certain behaviors reflect the cultural assumptions of the French physicians about the mentalities of the Senegalese. The cases of Moumar B. and Sihr B. exemplify the process of medicalization of religious experiences in a colonial context.

From the custodial hospital in Saint-Louis to the Saint-Pierre de Marseille asylum

Given the small numbers of mental patients, the authorities in Saint-Louis did not see the need for building an asylum. So the Civilian Hospital also served as a custodial hospital for the native insane, while the Military Hospital received the colonists. The evidence suggests that in the 1890s the hospital was in a deplorable situation. It did not have enough rooms to accommodate all the patients nor did it have in-patient psychiatric services.

This situation probably explains the authorities' willingness to return harmless mental patients to their families if the latter could promise in writing to watch the former and to take responsibility for their actions.[44] Parents and relatives of the patients took advantage of these provisions and petitioned the administration for the discharge of their relatives. But the authorities also recognized that the Civilian Hospital was not equipped to meet the medical needs of the insane, and there were no effective cures and remedies for most diseases.

The project to build an asylum in Saint-Louis was discussed and abandoned. In late 1890, Dr. Duval recommended the transfer of the insane to Cadillac (France) for humanitarian reasons as well as for economic considerations, given that the cost per patient per day (2 francs) was cheaper and the number of days of treatment fewer than in Senegal. He argued that the benefits of the transfer outweighed the rigor of French winters.[45] But a few months later, Dr. Carpot, a member of another powerful *métis* family, opposed this initiative, which he found "inefficient." "How can you believe," he wrote, "that people with incomplete cerebral organization, the maniacs and the melancholic, could change their lifestyle overnight?" The Interior Director also favored the status quo, and recommended the construction of an asylum in Saint-Louis but, if that was not possible, he was prepared to support the decision to transfer patients to Algeria or the Caribbean (Guadeloupe and Martinique).[46] The Colonial Commission also examined the same transfer proposal,[47] but reports from Paris indicated that there were no asylums in Algeria, and that the authorities in Guadeloupe and Martinique sent their insane to Saint-Morre de l'Assomption, Clermont Ferrand, or to the Saint-Pierre de Marseille Asylum, while the insane from Reunion Island were sent to Cadillac in Gironde (France) for the cost of 1.95 francs per patient per day.[48] No decision was made and the status quo remained.

As time went on, the combination of pressures from the patients' relatives and the increasing difficulties physicians faced in coping with overcrowding forced other administration officials to re-examine the question of transfer of the insane to better-equipped places within the French empire. Indeed, there were reports that some insane patients were discharged from the Civilian Hospital as cured and released back into the city, although they were still "absolutely dangerous" to their community. For example, merchants from Tivaouane complained that Sara D., who was discharged from the hospital, "was not cured but [only] mentally improved," and that she posed a serious danger of setting fire to their property.[49] So the authorities discussed again the question of the transfer of patients to alternative locations. Their choice fell on Marseille.

This decision did not please everyone, however. The *Médecin en Chef* formulated specific objections to it. From his perspective, the fact that the patients were illiterate in French was likely to make it difficult for them to communicate with the medical staff. His objections were also based on religious considerations, for he argued that it would be impossible for the Muslim patients to practice their religion, to perform funerary rites in case of death, or to observe dietary restrictions, such as the prohibition to eat pork. Even the imposition of the dress code, which required the compulsory adoption of the asylum uniform, was seen as a potential source of conflict.[50] But the Interior Director rejected the objections presented by the *Médecin en Chef*; he contended that one of the patients understood French and could be an interpreter between doctors and patients, that religious practices or dress code were of little use for the mentally deranged, and that they could avoid pork and wine.[51] Eventually, the *Conseil Privé*, in June 1897, approved the treaty that allowed the transfer of the insane to the Saint-Pierre de Marseille Public Asylum.[52] The administration officials still had to justify to themselves and to Paris the wisdom of the expenses to be engaged in the transfer of the native insane to France, in the light of Senegal's continuing financial crisis. Indeed, the minimum cost of health care in Marseille was estimated at 1.80 to 2 francs per patient per day. To address those concerns, the Interior Director underlined the absence of cure in Saint-Louis:

> Our doctors do not have at their disposal either the facilities, or the methods of treatment, or anything that would be necessary to provide efficient care to mental patients, ... the administration communicates with you in the hope that our patients would be put in normal conditions and would receive the intelligent and attentive care that you provide your patients.[53]

Indeed, the available treatment included the "use of mild tonics and sedatives, dietary restrictions and supplements, massages, low-current electrical stimulation, and visits to water spas and other health resorts."[54] Fully aware of the limits of the official medicine, the Interior Director underlined the altruistic character of the transfer operation by claiming that the administration was simply pursuing a "humanitarian objective,"[55] a "charity deed" (*l'oeuvre de pitié*), and he acknowledged that both the financial situation of Senegal and the small number of patients did not warrant the creation of an asylum. But he went beyond practical considerations to make a statement about the French perception of "Black Islam" (*Islam Noir*):

> These patients are Muslim but their Islamism, like that of most Negroes, is reduced to some external practices, such as the Salam, that can be performed anywhere and does not require the intervention of a clergy. At the hospice where they stay, they attend no religious ceremony.[56]

The Interior Director expressed the hope that the Director of the Saint-Pierre de Marseille Public Asylum would provide assistance.[57] Once the transfer decision was made, finding a carrier revealed more difficult. The *Société Générale de Transports Maritimes à Vapeur* flatly declined the offer made by the Interior Director. Finally, the deal was made with Fraissinet & Cie.[58] Following the agreement, cohorts of mental patients were sent to Marseille for health care. Yena A., who was among the first group of six men and five women to be transferred to Marseille, never made it to the destination; she died in transit, at Las Palmas.

The transfer of patients to Marseille created new problems for the asylum authorities. The fact that patients from Senegal did not speak nor understand French made it difficult to identify them simply on the basis of their file cases and in the absence of physical characteristics.[59] In addition, climatic changes combined with culture shock took their toll on the health of the transferred patients. Within a year of their arrival, Fatimata M. succumbed to pulmonary phthisis.[60] In contrast, Seck C., a twenty-eight-year-old mechanic, exhibited "notable improvement" and requested to be sent back to Senegal after a year of treatment.[61] Further research is needed to analyze the medical outcomes of the remaining transferred patients by using detailed, individual case reports.

Conclusion

The transformation of madness into a medical problem, in the absence of an asylum in Saint-Louis, created new challenges for the French colonial administration; it resulted in the sequestration of those the police classified as *aliéné(e)s*, or insane. The decision to transfer the native insane to France could be interpreted in the context of the rhetoric of the *mission civilisatrice* as a face-saving measure, at the time when the warehousing of the insane and the chronically ill, as well as the lack of funds to build a lunatic asylum, became a matter of acute embarrassment to colonial authorities. Colonial officials had all along emphasized the superiority of Western medicine over indigenous medicines, but in the cases of madness discussed here they were not able to produce evidence of its superiority. The discussions generated by the decision to transfer the native insane to France revealed the limits of republican universalism.

Notes

[1] "Ballacey to Prosecutor of the Republic, March 12, 1892," Archives Nationales du Sénégal (ANS)/H45/Sénégal.

[2] "Prosecutor General to Interior Director, July 12, 1897," ANS/H45/Sénégal.

[3] ANS/H45/Sénégal, "Prosecutor of Republic to General Prosecutor," no. 160, July 12, 1897.

[4] Treaty with Sénégal, Archives Départementales des Bouches-du-Rhone, Dossier 5 X 152. The treaty was due for renewal for nine years on May 5, 1906. See "Director of the Marseille Public Asylum for Insane to Préfet des Bouches-du-Rhone," Jan. 31, 1906, approving the renewal of the treaty.

[5] "État nominatif des aliénés placés d'office maintenues au 1er juillet 1904," Archives Départementales des Bouches du Rhone, Dossier 5 x 24, Asile Public d'Aliénés de Marseille, Section Hommes.

[6] Megan Vaughan, "Idioms of Madness: Zomba Lunatic Asylum, Nyasaland, in the Colonial Period," *Journal of Southern African Studies* 9 (1983): 218-38; Megan Vaughan, *Curing Their Ills: Colonial Power and African Illness* (Stanford: Stanford University Press, 1991), chap. 5.

[7] Jock McCulloch, *Colonial Psychiatry and the African Mind* (Cambridge: Cambridge University Press, 1995); Jock McCulloch, "The Theory and Practice of European Psychiatry in Colonial Africa," in *Colonialism and Psychiatry*, ed. Dinesh Bhugra and Roland Littlewood (New Delhi: Oxford University Press, 2001), 77-104.

[8] Jonathan Sadowsky, *Imperial Bedlam: Institutions of Madness in Colonial Southwest Nigeria* (University of California Press, 1999).

[9] Jonathan Sadowsky, "Confinement and Colonialism in Nigeria," in *The Confinement of the Insane: International Perspectives, 1850-1965*, ed. Roy Porter and David Wright (Cambridge: Cambridge University Press, 2003), 299.

[10] Harriett Deacon, "Insanity, Institutions and Society: the Case of the Robben Island Lunatic Asylum, 1846-1910," in *The Confinement of the Insane*, 20.

[11] Andrew Scull, *The Insanity of Place/The Place of Insanity. Essays on the History of Psychiatry* (New York: Routledge, 2006), 4-8, 41; See also Andrew Scull, "The Frail

Foundations of Foucault's Monument," *The Times Literary Supplement*, March 23, 2007: 3-4; Colin Gordon, "In Defence of Foucault," *The Times Literary Supplement*, April 6, 2007: 3; Andrew Scull, "Foucault and Madness," *The Times Literary Supplement*, April 20, 2007: 15.

[12] James H. Mills, *Madness, Canabis and Colonialism. The 'Native-Only' Lunatic Asylums of British Inida, 1857-1900* (New York: Saint-Martin's Press, Inc., 2000), 3.

[13] Shula Marks, "'Every Facility That Modern Science and Enlightened Humanity Have Devised': Race and Progress in a Colonial Hospital," in *Insanity, Institutions and Society, 1800-1914: A Social History of Madness in Comparative Perspective*, ed. Joseph Melling and Bill Forsythe (New York: Routledge, 1999), 268-91; Vaughan, *Curing their Ills*.

[14] Roy Porter, introduction to Sadowsky, *The Confinement of the Insane*, 4.

[15] Mills, *Madness, Canabis and Colonialism*, 2.

[16] Mamadou Diouf and Mohamed Mboj, "L'administration coloniale et la question de l'aliénation mentale (1840-1956)," in *La folie au Sénégal*, ed. Ludovic d'Almeida et al (Dakar : ACS, 1997), 13-54.

[17] "Director of the Civilian Hospital to Interior Director," no.1, Jan.19, 1891, ANS/-H102/Sénégal.

[18] French doctors used the terms "alienation mentale" and "affections mentales," not "psychiatrie."

[19] Mamadou Diouf and Mohamed Mbodj, "L'administration coloniale et la question de l'aliénation mentale (1840-1956)," 19-21.

[20] "Procureur de la République to Procureur Général," no.719, July 12, 1897, ANS/-H45/Sénégal. See also the article 489 of the Code Civil.

[21] "Jules B. to Interior Director," February 1, 1898, ANS/H45/Sénégal.

[22] "Médecin en Chef to Governor General of French West Africa," no.275, Sept. 14, 1897, ANS/H9/188.

[23] "Médecin en Chef to Governor General of French West Africa," no.134, April 19, 1897, ANS/H9/AOF/183.

[24] Michel Foucault, *Discipline and Punish* (Harmmondsworth, 1979).

[25] "Médecin en Chef to Interior Director," no.301, February 4, 1898, ANS/H45/Sénégal.

[26] "Nisolation," instead of "isolation," in this passage, was probably a typo, since in the same letter Camille also used "isolation."

[27] "Camille R. to the Minister of Colonies," April 25, 1898, ANS/H45/Sénégal.

[28] Ann Braden Johnson, *Out of Bedlam: The Truth About De-Institutionalization* (Boston: Basic Books, 1990), 112, cited by Jonathan Sadowsky, *Imperial Bedlam*, 50.

[29] "B. to ?," April 12, 1897, ANS/H45/Sénégal.

[30] "B. to the Prosecutor of the Republic," June 21, 1897, ANS/H45/Sénégal.

[31] "Billet d'Admission du Bureau des Entrées, Asile d'Aliénés de Marseille," March 25, 1898, ANS/H45/Sénégal., recording B., married, French, former administrator, aged thirty-eight years, arriving from Senegal. This is a case file for Jules B.; the incidents described allegedly took place between 1895 and 1897.

[32] "Ballacey to Prosecutor of the Republic," March 12, 1892, ANS/H45/Sénégal.

[33] "Camille R. to Minister of Colonies," April 25, 1898, ANS/H45/Sénégal.

[34] "Billet d'Admission du Bureau des Entrées," note 22 above.

[35] After his deportation to Gabon (1895-7) and Mauritania (1903-7), the French realized that Ahmadou Bamba's doctrine of hard work actually served French interests. Also,

he helped the French authorities recruit Senegalese troops for the First World War, an effort that prompted the authorities to grant him a Légion d'Honneur medal.

[36] "Ballacey to Prosecutor of the Republic," March 12, 1892, ANS/H45/Sénégal.

[37] "B. to Interior Director," July 23, 1898, ANS/H45/Sénégal.

[38] "Director of the Marseille Asylum to the Interior Director of Senegal," no. 1387, March 24, 1898, ANS/H45/Sénégal.

[39] "Director of Civilian Hospital to Interior Director," no.1, January 19, 1891, ANS/H102/Sénégal.

[40] "Administrator of Tivaouane to Director of Indigenous Affairs," no. 679, September 28, 1898; "Director of Indigenous Affairs to Administrator of Tivaouane," official cable, September 28, 1898; "General Prosecutor to Secretary General of Government," September 29, 1898; "Chief Commissar Aubry Lecomte to Police Commissar," note related to Moumar Diakhate, October 1898. All in ANS/H45/Sénégal.

[41] "Dr. Henry Reboul to Colonel Commandant Supérior des Troupes," no. 96 of April 11, 1897, ANS/H9/AOF/185; "Medical certificate of madness, April 11, 1897," ANS/H9/AOF/186.

[42] "General Prosecutor to General Secretary of Government," no. 189 of Sept. 29, 1898; "Official cable from the Director of Indigenous Affairs to the Administrator of Tivaouane," Sept. 28, 1898; "Deputy Director of Indigenous Affairs to General Prosecutor," Sept. 28, 1898. All in ANS/H45/Sénégal.

[43] Dr. Pelletier's observations, April 2, 1908, and "Boubacar to Governor," n.d., ANS/H54/Sénégal.

[44] "Charles Legros to Chief of Staff of General Secretary," Dec. 21, 1898, ANS/H45/Sénégal.

[45] "Dr. Duval to Interior Director," no. 89 of Nov. 25, 1890, ANS/H45/Sénégal.

[46] "Dr. Carpot to Interior Director," June 15, 1891, ANS/H45/Sénégal.

[47] Colonial Commission meeting records, June 22, 1891, ANS/H45/Sénégal.

[48] "1ère Division 1er Bureau (Paris) to governor of Senegal," no. 53 of Aug. 17, 1891, ANS/H45/Sénégal.

[49] "Administrator of Tivaouane Galibert to Interior Delegate in Dakar," Jan. 21, 1896, ANS/H45/Sénégal.

[50] "Director of the Marseille Asylum to Interior Director," no. 678 of Jan. 12, 1897, ANS/H45/Sénégal.

[51] Ibid., annotations on the margin of the letter.

[52] "2e Bureau to Interior Director, June 8, 1897.

[53] "Interior Director of Senegal to the Saint-Pierre de Marseille Public Asylum," no. 27, January 28, 1898, and "Director of the Saint-Pierre de Marseille Public Asylum to Interior Director of Senegal," no. 1387 of March 24, 1898, ANS/H45/Sénégal.

[54] Jack D. Pressman, "Concepts of Mental Illness in the West," in *The Cambridge World History of Human Disease*, ed. Kenneth F. Kipple (New York: Cambridge University Press, 1993), 72.

[55] "Director of the Marseille Asylum to Interior Director," no. 678, Jan. 12, 1897, annotations on the margin of the letter, ANS/H45/Sénégal.

[56] "Interior Director of Senegal to the Saint-Pierre de Marseille Public Asylum," no. 27 of January 28, 1898, and "Director of the Saint-Pierre de Marseille Public Asylum to

Interior Director of Senegal," no. 1387 of March 24, 1898, ANS/H45/Sénégal.

[57] Ibid.

[58] "Fraissinet & Cie Agent to the Interior Director," no. 569 of June 13, 1897, ANS/H45/Sénégal.

[59] "Director of Saint-Pierre de Marseille Public Asylum to Interior Director of Senegal," no. 1387 of March 24, 1898, ANS/H45/Sénégal.

[60] "Death certificate," no. 5868, July 13, 1898, ANS/H45/Sénégal.

[61] Police Records, December 20, 1898, ANS/H45/Sénégal.

CHAPTER 11

Commodity *Fetichismo*, the Holy Spirit, and the Turn to Pentecostal and African Independent Churches in Central Mozambique[1]

JAMES PFEIFFER

Introduction

Pentecostals and African Independent Churches (AICs) influenced by Pentecostalism have rapidly spread throughout central Mozambique in the aftermath of war and in the midst of a structural adjustment program that has hastened commoditization of community life and intensified local inequalities over the last decade. The AICs, which include "Zionist" and "Apostolic" movements (the AICs) from South Africa and Zimbabwe, have found fertile ground for growth among the poor, who are recruited primarily through healing. Other churches more directly identified as Pentecostal, including various manifestations of the Assemblies of God, the Apostolic Faith Mission, Universal Church-Kingdom of God, and the Full Gospel Church have had similar success in attracting new members through healing.[2] The extraordinary expansion of these movements in Mozambique signals a dramatic and important shift away from reliance on "traditional" healers, known as *nyanga* or *n'anga* in Shona dialects and *curandeiros* in Portuguese, to treat persistent afflictions believed to have spiritual causes. As argued elsewhere by the author,[3] the popularity of the churches has in part been driven by growing inequality in the last decade that may have heightened perceived spiritual threats to health and good fortune in an environment of deepening insecurity and conflict. Based on more recent illness narrative interviews of church recruits in the central Mozambican city of Chimoio, the current article focuses more specifically on how curandeiros have increased fees and tailored treatments to clients searching for good fortune in ways that have alienated many other help seekers in this social environment.

Fees have risen in the context of widening local economic disparities, creating further social dilemmas for clients seeking new prosperity or combating persistent misfortunes in the form of illness, infertility, job loss, financial struggles, or familial conflict. The higher cost of traditional treatment in itself is a barrier to consulting curandeiros for many of the poor. But equally important is how the inflation of fees in the context of increasingly stark social inequalities taints the legitimacy of the therapeutic process itself by eroding trust and confidence and introducing skepticism into patient-healer interactions. While traditional healing has been celebrated and even romanticized in the international health world, community attitudes toward curandeiros are decidedly less generous, and their healing activities are increasingly viewed with suspicion because of their engagement with often malevolent and frightening occult forces used to foment social conflict, competition, and confrontation. The conspicuous sale of curandeiro services for high profit appears to be one of the most troubling aspects of traditional healing for many help seekers in this environment; access to these occult forces is being sold at elevated prices to enrich the provider, often at great expense and danger to others. In contrast, the churches' healing approach emphasizes a less divisive and more pervasive spiritual protection offered without payment and reinforced by social support in a new collectivity. It is argued here that one vital source of the movement's recent popularity derives from church efforts to promote this contrast and effectively exploit the already considerable community anxiety over rising curandeiro fees and their socially divisive treatments in an increasingly insecure environment.

This expansion of churches in Mozambique parallels similar growth of Pentecostal and AIC movements across the continent, especially southern Africa, in recent years. The critical role of healing to this expansion is well-documented, and the churches' success within urbanizing communities is believed by many to derive, at least in part, from how they soothe the trauma of social dislocation, dispersion, and "anomie" in the transition to modernity.[4] Healing practices, especially among AICs, are reported to be "syncretistic" in their incorporation of local idioms of social distress and illness causation related to this transition. Earlier explanations for Pentecostal popularity in Africa focused on this healing syncretism that was thought to provide a "bridge" back to tradition for disoriented and nostalgic urban migrants bewildered by their new circumstances.[5] Later explanations centered on whether church popularity represented "resistance" or "acquiescence" to European domination and the political economy of apartheid.[6] In the post-colonial and post-apartheid period, a new paradigm of sorts has emerged that locates AIC and Pentecostal success within the globalization and transition to modernity problematic by emphasizing church rejection of "tradition" as a "break with the past," an embrace of modernity, and participation in a new social identity that transcends ethnicity and nation.[7] To join these movements, members break with their individual pasts, represented by ties to family and tradition in rural areas, to create a new, modern, urban, more individual subject freed from the constraints of rural family demands and backward beliefs.[8] In this view, traditional healers are often vilified and demonized by Pentecostal movements primarily because they are "traditional" and therefore believed to keep individuals mired in backwardness and poverty, impeding progress toward modernity and prosperity.[9]

The illness narratives described here, which focus on lay member patterns of health-seeking that preceded and motivated the turn to prophet-healers, tend, however, to provide conversion stories that do not fit well within this new paradigm. While "demonization" of traditional healers by Pentecostals is widely reported, there is little available in the current literature that explains why this demonization resonates so strongly among so many of the poor, and why local healers should lose their legitimacy and perceived efficaciousness in treating the same illness-causing spiritual afflictions and occult threats that prophet-healers address. In these narratives, church members speak less of rejecting the past than of their disillusionment with the intensified commodification of traditional healing in a changing social environment of sharpening income disparities and declining social security: an environment generated in part by economic liberalization and structural adjustment over the last decade.

Traditional healing practices have increasingly been tailored and sold to men who often pay high fees to practice, or protect against, sorcery related to obtaining employment or undermining competitors. As the market has grown for these kinds of curandeiro services in the struggle to obtain scarce urban jobs amidst the lure of potential wealth in the growing economy, treatments for maternal and child health complaints have been priced out of many women's range. A majority of women cannot pay for curandeiro treatments themselves. Although church explanatory models for illness incorporate many of the same local Shona idioms of social distress deployed by traditional healers, pastors and prophets have imported the Pentecostal notion of the universal "Holy Spirit" (*Mwiya Mutsene* in Chiteve, and *Espirito Santo* in Portuguese) to provide broad protection for free against relentless occult threats to health and well-being emanating from the deeply conflictive social environment.

Most respondents recounted long, frustrating periods of seeking help from various sources, including biomedical providers, home remedies, black market pharmaceuticals, and curandeiros, often simultaneously, before finally turning to church prophets, usually in desperation to resolve a persistent affliction. Often, disparate episodes of illness and misfortune among different family members, especially children, are woven together to reveal the intervention of a "bad spirit," or *espirito mau* in Portuguese. However, as many of the stories unfold, more nuanced accounts reveal that traditional healers came to be perceived as ineffective and distrusted not because they offered traditional remedies, but rather because of the inflation of their fees in the sale of services as commodities through which the healers themselves often gain conspicuous wealth. It is not argued here that commodification of traditional healing is something new; curandeiros have reportedly been "paid" in some form or another for many years in Mozambique. Rather, economic disparity has increased so rapidly that rising fees for curandeiro services have become suspect within this changing social environment, where "everyone is out for themselves" [*cada um para cada um* in Portuguese], in the words of one informant. The circulation of money and the commodification of treatment have new effects and have taken on new meaning in an environment in which the social gradient has steepened so quickly. Many curandeiros are perceived to be complicit in advancing their clients' fortunes at the expense of others, all while profiting themselves. In the current context characterized by both increasing social and geographic mobility, curandeiros can cause conflicts within families or between neighbors and co-workers to spin disastrously out of control. Many of those interviewed turned to, and trusted, church prophet-healers in part because treatment for the same spiritual afflictions did not inflame these conflicts.

In direct contrast to the inflating curandeiro fees, church treatments are not "purchased," and the lack of payment is cited by help-seekers as an indication of both authenticity and good intentions. Financial contributions to churches are vitally important, but not linked to treatments, as discussed below in more detail. Pastors and prophets are keenly aware of the ambivalence felt by many toward curandeiros and emphatically stress that the Holy Spirit is an entirely different healing power in continual struggle with the harmful occult forces that traditional healers engage. Since church healers ply the same spiritual terrain as local curandeiros, often exorcizing malevolent spirits using local terms and idioms, drawing this distinction becomes especially critical to attracting new members. The contrast between the sale of curandeiro services and the churches' offer of free healing provides just the opportunity to tap into deepening local anxieties about new forms of accumulation, growing social competition, and importance of access to cash for survival in the commoditizing economy. Rapidly widening disparities, and alleged curandeiro complicity in generating new inequalities, have brought this contrast into even sharper relief, and churches have used it effectively to undermine curandeiro legitimacy in the eyes of many.

Healing, Witchcraft, and Inequality

In both the old and new literature on "witchcraft," the term is used broadly to encompass a range of practices related to the occult that often include healing.[10] Traditional healing in most southern Africa societies can involve activities that fall under the rubric of "witchcraft" more broadly. Given the nature of their skills, curandeiros can potentially harness both the positive and destructive powers of the spirit world, that is, the volatile world of the dead, to cure, bring good luck, send misfortune, or kill. The confusion concerning the relationship and overlap among witchcraft, sorcery, and healing practices reflects the ambivalence that many in Chimoio feel about curandeiros. Geschiere describes a similar ambivalence in Cameroon, where he has analyzed court cases involving accusations of witchcraft.[11]

> Indeed, an accused who dares to call himself a *sorcier* is sure to be put in jail. Yet the *nganga* [healer] does so without any further reaction from the judges. Apparently the latter recognize that there are different types of *sorciers*, some of which have to be punished, while others (the *nganga*) are valuable allies in the struggle against *la sorcellerie*. This terminological confusion has deeper implications. Officially, the State and its servants condemn witchcraft as an evil,

to be eradicated altogether. Privately, however, many civil servants (judges included) are deeply involved with witchcraft, enlisting the services of *nganga* to protect them or even to attack their rivals. The murderous competition for posts and promotion in the public service is a hotbed for witchcraft rumours and machinations.

The fact that occult practices, including healing and sorcery, help individuals manage these kinds of new inequalities has attracted a renewed interest in "witchcraft" among anthropologists.[12] As Geschiere has emphasized, witchcraft can be both a leveling force, undermining inequalities in wealth and power, but also instrumental for individual accumulation and social mobility. He writes, "Witchcraft is both jealousy and success. It is used to kill but also to heal."[13] Classic anthropology on witchcraft and sorcery emphasized the integration of occult practices with local dynamics of "envy," notions of "the limited good," misfortune, and good fortune.[14] Whether in its power of explanation or in its instrumentality, witchcraft has provided a lens to interpret inequalities that both disrupt and animate social life. And, as Jean and John Comaroff emphasize, "[W]itchcraft is not simply an imaginative 'idiom.' It is chillingly concrete, its micropolitics all-too-real. As Evans-Pritchard (1937) long ago maintained, its occurrence is explicable only with reference to its particular pragmatics; to the ways in which, in specific contexts, it permits the allocation of responsibility for, and demands action upon, palpable human inequities and misfortunes."[15] Much of the new literature argues that modernity has not brought disenchantment as predicted by earlier Weberian theorists, but rather witchcraft and occult practices may be increasing in contemporary Africa, at least in part because of their usefulness in responding to new inequalities that emerge with modernity. As Moore and Sanders suggest, however, "[C]ontemporary scholars of witchcraft cast occult beliefs and practices as not only contiguous with, *but constitutive of modernity*."[16] Sanders specifically links the perceived expansion of these practices in Tanzania to recent economic reform, "[I]n the era of structural adjustment, the occult itself has been commodified and thus vastly expanded both in the popular imagination and its practical reach."[17]

The market for these kinds of services predictably grows as social insecurity is heightened and the healers themselves, who are usually very poor, have also found rewarding ways to ply their trade. Hence the purported increase in, or increased anxieties about, competitive and dangerous forms of sorcery purchased from curandeiros in communities like Chimoio. Poor women are at a special disadvantage in these circumstances since most are unable to generate any significant cash to pay for protective treatment, yet they remain in desperate need of spiritual defense given their reproductive roles amidst extraordinarily difficult material conditions and dwindling familial support.[18] The evidence presented here suggests that laymembers' decisions to seek help from churches and join these movements were not necessarily experienced as a break with tradition. Traditional healing practices had already themselves been transformed to address the afflictions of a "modernity" wrought by colonial penetration that has generated vast changes in social life and healing practices in the region for over a century. In this post-colonial and post-socialist moment, curandeiro practices have again adjusted to accommodate local fears and desires incited by "free markets" and state withdrawal. This adjustment is manifested in an emphasis on the sale of services most useful to individual enrichment at the expense of social competitors. Far from helping urban migrants to sever their rural family ties and embrace a new "modern" individuality, the churches appear to offer a new collectivity as an alternative to curandeiros/sorcerers who would otherwise foment social conflict and arouse dangerous occult powers for a high fee. In Chimoio, the flight to churches is as much a flight from the modernity of traditional healing as it is a break with the past.

Research Design and Methods

The interviews described here were collected as part of a larger study of AIC and Pentecostal expansion in Chimoio and of the relationship of that expansion to structural adjustment and deepening social inequality in the region. In addition to the collection of illness narratives, the research included a survey of three contiguous peri-urban *bairros* (or neighborhoods) selected for their large populations of residents representing a broad socioeconomic range with demographic similarity to the rest of the city. The population of the three *bairros* together totals over 21,000 people.[19] The survey of 616 men and women using systematic random sampling was conducted to identify the range of churches in the community, estimate the level of participation in each faith, gather demographic information, and measure social attitudes using a set of Likert-scale questions concerning perceptions of changes in social inequality, social well-being, occult practices, and access to basic services. The survey interviews each lasted about one hour.

Pastors from eight of the churches in the *bairros* helped to identify other men and women who were recent converts for more in-depth open-ended illness narrative interviews. These interviews focused on health-seeking decisions and experiences that led the respondents to seek help from the churches. Eighty illness narrative interviews were conducted in 2002 and 2003, and dozens of other similar interviews conducted in 1998 and 2000 in the same *bairros* were also re-analyzed in relationship to the central questions in the current research. An additional 30 interviews were conducted in 2003 with randomly selected *bairro* residents who were not church members to identify and contrast recent health-seeking patterns of resort, attitudes toward curandeiros, and opinions about church healers.

Chimoio in Transition

The population of Chimoio, the capital of Manica Province, has more than tripled since independence in 1975, expanding from about 50,000 to over 170,000 as thousands moved to the city in search of safety during the 15-year war with South Africa-backed rebels (known by their Portuguese acronym RENAMO) that ended in 1992. In order to survive the austerity economy, most Chimoio residents are peasant-proletarians who combine cash-earning opportunities with subsistence production, cultivating maize and sorghum outside the city on small parcels of land called *machambas*. Chimoio is a multi-lingual city where *Chiteve*, a variant in the *Shona*-based family of languages that extends across most of Zimbabwe and central Mozambique, is spoken by a majority. But a number of other Shona dialects and local languages are also heard, including *Chindau, Chisena, Chinhungwe, Shangana,* and *Tonga*. Portuguese is also widely used by most residents in this multilingual environment. Standard health indicators reveal the impact of severe material deprivation; cumulative under-five mortality is estimated at about 200/1000,[20] while maternal mortality was estimated at 1,500/100,000 for the entire country during this period.[21]

With affliction so common and unrelenting in this community, there are hundreds of curandeiros, both herbalists and spiritual healers, distributed throughout the city, who continue to be widely consulted. In Chimoio, the National Health Service (NHS) provides biomedical care through the provincial hospital, and at several health centers offering basic primary health care services distributed in other parts of the city. A private health clinic serving the small emerging elite that can afford the high fees opened in the city in the mid-1990s. While most state services are free or inexpensive, providers reportedly ask for under-the-table payments, a problem that worsened when health worker salaries dropped with economic adjustment.[22] Pharmaceuticals stolen from clinics and hospitals, including chloroquin and antibiotics, are widely available in outdoor markets or at private homes. The churches have now entered this already medically plural environment, some offering spiritual healing that incorporates local notions of illness and others practicing prayer healing and laying-on of hands.

The Church Expansion in Chimoio

According to the 1997 census, the Zion churches have become the largest religious category in urban areas in Manica Province, claiming about 30 percent of the population. Nearly five percent identified themselves as "Protestant/Evangelical," a category consisting mostly of Pentecostals.[23] It is likely that since census data were collected in the mid-1990s church participation expanded even further. Catholic Church membership declined from about 30 percent in the 1980 census to 20 percent in urban areas. In the current survey of three *bairros* reported here, nearly 45 percent of respondents belonged to churches described as Zionist, Apostolic, or Pentecostal. About 12 percent identified as Zionist, 13 percent belonged to Apostolic churches that use prophetic healing (and are often called Zionists by outsiders), and a further 20 percent were members of a wide range of Pentecostal churches. In just the three *bairros* surveyed here, over 40 distinctly named affiliations to which respondents belonged were identified within these three church groups. Catholics accounted for about 23 percent of the total sample. Gender differences in participation were evident as well. Nearly 16 percent of all women respondents were members of Zion churches in contrast to 8 percent of men. Twenty-two percent of women versus 17 percent of men belonged to Pentecostals, while nearly 26 percent of men were members of the Catholic Church in contrast to only 20 percent of women. By 2002, the Department of Religious Affairs registered over 200 individual AIC and Pentecostal variants in Chimoio, up from 30 in the early 1990s.

Rapid AIC and Pentecostal expansion in the 1990s also gained momentum in part because the Mozambican government loosened its regulation of religious expression, allowing church movements from the southern Africa region to enter Mozambique and proselytize more freely.[24] Since then, all churches have been able to recruit and mobilize members without the government interference and oversight that characterized the post-independence period in the 1970s and 1980s. The end of the war opened the region to greater movement and circulation of people and ideas while the economy was also being liberalized. Disentangling which of these historical factors contributed most to the dramatic growth of these religious movements is nearly impossible, and to argue, as some do in Mozambique, that Pentecostal growth is simply the result of this opening of society in the late 1980s fails to explain why the Pentecostalist wave grew so quickly while other equally repressed faiths dwindled. One can only speculate as to whether the Pentecostals would have expanded just as quickly during the socialist period if they had had freedom to proselytize. And the phenomenon is not restricted to Mozambique; similar and related movements have swept across other regions of Africa in recent years, further suggesting that more general social-historical processes may be implicated in growing church popularity. The narratives described here suggest that the striking economic changes of the 1990s that accelerated commoditization and increased inequality had a distinct role in church growth.

Adjustment

In 1987, these broad changes in social and economic life were introduced by a World Bank/IMF structural adjustment program (SAP) while the war still dragged on.[25] The SAP led to privatization, shredding of social safety nets, cutbacks in social services, arrival of foreign aid, and growing corruption that has spawned rapid class formation and glaring economic disparities over a very short period.[26] In the earlier years after independence, labor migration from the region to South Africa was also curtailed, eliminating an important source of income for some households, but significant male migration continued within the country and to Zimbabwe during and after the war. Social and economic changes accelerated further after the fighting ended in 1992, when economic activity could be conducted free from fear of attack. The change in social environment in local communities over this period cannot be overestimated. While Mozambique has been hailed for its relatively robust economic growth in the 1990s, benefits have trickled up to a small business elite while many Mozambicans remain mired in absolute poverty.[27] It has become an economy in which the attraction of wealth and goods flowing into the city is juxtaposed against deepened economic and social insecurity in a kind of austerity/luxury economy. Accumulation by the few is visible around the city, where hundreds of larger cement houses are under construction, satellite dishes and antennae have appeared on many homes, and expensive SUVs and private luxury cars cruise the streets. Even in poorer *bairros*, some have managed to obtain paying work with foreign aid agencies or local businesses and to build new cement houses. One wealthy area of the city became known as the *"bairro dos ladrões"* (neighborhood of thieves, i.e. the corrupt) in the 1990s and later *"bairro dos cabritos,"* literally neighborhood of the goats, after President Joaquim Chissano suggested in a national radio address that corrupt bureaucrats were like tethered goats that eat everything within their reach. *Cabritismo* (literally goatism) has become the central metaphor for corruption in national discourse.

In the eyes of many, the new conspicuous consumption and wealth in the city appears to have no visible source or explanation; new wealth is often assumed to be obtained through crime, corruption, or practice of sorcery capabilities purchased from corrupt curandeiros. Likert scale data in the survey for this research revealed that over 80 percent of respondents either agreed somewhat or agreed strongly that since the war's end only a few had gotten wealthier while most people had gotten poorer. Nearly 45 percent of respondents felt that their own households had gotten poorer since the war's end, while only 30 percent felt that they had gotten wealthier.

The expanded trade of sexual favors for money or goods is another product of the deepened social inequality that has undermined economic security for many women. These activities range from full time sex work around neighborhood bars to casual provision of sexual favors in exchange for cash or goods such as shoes or clothing. Likert scale data on the survey revealed that over 80 percent of respondents believed that prostitution and promiscuity (roughly translated as *curtição* locally) had increased over the previous 10-year period; nearly 68 percent believed it had increased a great deal. The resulting pressure on intrahousehold relationships has produced greater distrust, allegations of adultery, and fear of the spread of sexually transmitted infections including, of course, AIDS. The ensuing moral panic in Chimoio has not only destabilized relationships, families, and households, it has also generated a backlash within the churches against condom promotion campaigns that are seen as encouraging promiscuity and prostitution.

This is not to suggest that social life in the region had not already been directly integrated into market relationships for at least a century, if not longer. Large-scale male labor migration to Southern Rhodesia, South Africa, and local plantations, in addition to participation in local trading, had long been the social and economic reality for Mozambicans under Portuguese rule. Bridewealth, known locally as *lobolo*, has long been paid in cash in the area, and cash payment to curandeiros has reportedly been common for some time, especially in towns and cities. The socialist period after independence certainly curtailed market activities, but money was still exchanged for a variety of services and goods. The recent period of free market promotion and privatization, however, marks an especially intense deepening of the commoditization of social life and associated social differentiation. As the cash price of *lobolo* has inflated, many men can no longer pay, and choose to live with their partners without formal marriage status. In this survey, over 50 percent reported that they lived with a partner but were not married. Many informants remarked that ceremonies to clear *machambas* based on mutual reciprocity were maintained well into the recent war years, but with economic adjustment nearly everyone now demands cash payment to work for others. Much of the land for *machambas* and matoros was formerly allocated by local *regulos*, or chiefs known as *mambos* in Shona, based on local notions of justice and kin-based land rights. The socialist period saw the state assume many of these functions, especially in the creation of state farms and communal villages. But in the post-war period of adjustment, small farmers increasingly have had to rent or pay for their land in spite of new land tenure laws. As food subsidies have been eliminated, and fees (both legal and illegal) for health and education have been introduced, cash income has become increasingly crucial to survival for the vulnerable, and to social mobility for the ambitious.[28]

The deepened commodification of so many aspects of social life has occurred simultaneously with, and has helped to cause, rapid class formation and conspicuous accumulation of a fortunate few. Of course, sharp social disparities are not new in a region whose recent history is defined by the severe inequalities of Portuguese rule. What distinguishes the current period from both the socialist and colonial epochs is not simply commoditization and the arrival of modernity (both had already happened in some form or other in Chimoio) but rather the rapid *increase* in new local inequalities based primarily on access to cash, and marked by intensified economic insecurity for some and new wealth for others in a sink or swim market. In this environment, the desperate need for money has superseded and in some ways dissolved previous social obligations, family relationships, and other sources of reciprocity and support, beyond the conventional notions of urban "anomie" and social disruption associated with the general processes of migration and urbanization that characterize modernity in the Third World.

In this environment, the high price of curandeiro services has an especially important impact on women, most of whom have little or no cash income of their own. In the survey here, nearly 60 percent of women stated that they had earned no cash income at all in the previous month, in contrast to only 10 percent of men who earned none. While 52 percent of men earned over 500,000 *meticais* (24,000 *meticais* to one US dollar) in the previous month, only 13 percent of women earned in that range. Previous research in a nearby community also demonstrated that men and women normally control separate income streams within households, so that the many women who do not earn their own money can only use cash at the behest of their husbands. They must decide whether to risk asking a spouse for money to treat an affliction believed to derive from intrahousehold conflict or familial discord. Indeed, most women reported consulting curandeiros only with spouses or family members, in part so they can pay. In contrast, most women reported seeking help from prophets on their own since cash payment was not necessary; later they often attempted to bring their partners into the church.[29]

Spirits, Inequality, and Sorcery in an Age of Adjustment

Traditional healing in this region of Mozambique, specifically "therapy" that engages the spirit/occult world, involves attempts to influence spiritual forces believed to underlie fortune and misfortune, including illness. In this complex and intricate moral universe, both extraordinary fortune and misfortune can be viewed suspiciously. Sorcery, vengeful spirits, angry

ancestral spirits, and "immoral" behavior such as infidelity are often implicated in experiences of misfortune, including health problems, but spirits
can also be manipulated and mobilized for personal gain.[30] When illness is
accompanied by unusual symptoms or circumstances, or when biomedical
interventions fail, a spiritual cause might be considered and a curandeiro
consulted to exorcise the offending spirits and provide continued protection.
On the other hand, someone who is especially successful and accumulates
material wealth and power may also be suspected of engaging the occult
world, with the help of a curandeiro, for self-promotion and perhaps to
harm social competitors.

The English term *witchcraft* conflates diverse modalities of engagement
with the spirit world and translations into Portuguese or Chiteve create
further ambiguities and qualifications. In Chimoio, dangerous occult practices are roughly divided into two categories of practitioners and activities
that resonate quite differently in the new social environment. The Chiteve
term *uroyi*, and in Portuguese *feitiço*, or *wakoroya* (or *varoya*) in Chiteve
and *feiticeiro/as* in Portuguese, is often used in reference to the activity
of "witches," who are women born with an inherited malevolent spirit that
can cause terrible misfortune. In contrast, "sorcery" abilities are purchased
from curandeiros and are practiced through use of special substances that
can harm one's enemies or provide good fortune. Health metaphors are embedded in the Portuguese terms employed for "treatment" of a wide range
of life problems by sorcery practices using these substances and spiritual
powers. *Kukamba* and *kurom* are Chiteve terms for the purchase of sorcery powers from curandeiros activated through substances called *mutombo*
in Chiteve and translated as *medicamentos* (medicines) or *drogas* (drugs)
in Portuguese. The Portuguese term *medicamentos da vida* is often used
to distinguish *mutombo* that will help a man obtain employment or other
good fortune outside the realm of biomedical health, narrowly defined. But
the terms *medicamentos* or *mutombo* are also used in practices that harm
others, that is, to send sickness or misfortune. The Portuguese term *feitiço*,
or sometimes *fetichismo*, is also heard in reference to this kind of sorcery
activity, but a second Portuguese term, *drogar* (literally "to use drugs") is
more common to distinguish it from *uroyi*, or the activity of witches.

The distinction between *feiticeiro/as* and *drogados* emerged clearly in
several questions on social attitudes in the survey for this research. The
survey asked respondents separate questions concerning whether *feitiço*

and *drogados* had increased or decreased over the previous ten-year period. Over 64 percent responded that the use of "drogas" had increased, and over 42 percent agreed that it had increased a great deal. In contrast, nearly 42 percent believed that the problem of witches had actually diminished and only 36 percent believed it had increased at all. In pretests of the survey instrument, respondents clearly distinguished between the two kinds of activity. The practice of *kukamba* or *kuromba* for protection, good luck, or social aggression constitutes a key set of practices in the curandeiro's treatment repertoire that might be called witchcraft in English but is distinct from the practice of "witches," or wakoroya, in Chimoio. The survey findings suggest that occult practices that can be bought and sold in the new economy are the ones perceived to have increased in the new economic and social environment. Analysis of the survey data also suggests that the perception of increased use of "drogas" is broadly shared among church and non-church respondents.

The exchange of money and the high prices of curandeiro services are also linked to an aura of danger surrounding many consultations. Tales abound of corrupt healers who charge outrageous fees, engage in sorcery to harm others or promote good fortune, and enrich themselves by fomenting conflict within families and among neighbors. Treatments can involve an inversion of the moral world in which help-seekers are required to engage in reprehensible activities such as sleeping with one's mother or daughter, necrophilia, or taking a life to secure occult powers of protection and enrichment. Acts of moral abomination are one source of occult power and require tremendous courage on the part of the help-seeker. The greater the risk taken, the greater the potential pay-off. The demons that are mobilized in these treatment processes are unpredictable, unstable, and extremely dangerous. Paying a curandeiro to engage this world to provide protection, gain good fortune, or harm one's social enemies can go wildly wrong and result in a descent into madness for the help-seeker or misfortune for one's family. "Drogas" gone wrong is the most common explanation for the many mentally ill men who now wander the streets of Chimoio in rags. Curandeiros are sometimes implicated in the startling increase in crime that began after the war's end in the region. One frequently mentioned activity involves paying a fee to a corrupt curandeiro who helps the client steal water used to wash corpses in the city mortuary. The water, with its spiritual power, can be ritually treated by the curandeiro to obtain the effect of putting victims to sleep temporarily when it is sprinkled around their home at night. Thieves can then break in and steal everything while the occupants are unconscious. They awake in the morning to see all their possessions taken, but have heard nothing since they had been drugged.

As described elsewhere, curandeiros function within a complex spirit world that requires some brief description. Ancestral guardian spirits, *w(v)adzimu* in Chiteve (or *midzimu* in other Shona dialects), can provide protection from spiritual threats and should be honored regularly, usually through ritual beer brewing and festivities.[31] Severe illness caused by malevolent spirits and sorcery can result from ancestors' withdrawal of protection for failure to follow ritual patterns of respect, "immoral" behavior such as infidelity, and intrafamily conflict. In Chimoio, avenging spirits of murder victims are among the most dangerous since they seek revenge by creating illness, misfortune or death in the murderer's family.[32] Intrafamily conflict and tension is also often attributed to the presence of such avenging spirits, which are called *mupfukwa* in Chimoio. Such spirits can also be aroused with the help of a curandeiro by a family seeking to avenge the murder of a relative or to enforce the return of stolen property or payment of debt.

Spirits of both affliction and healing often emanate from important historical periods and events in the social history of a region. Curandeiros and prophet-healers both spoke of the spirits of Gungunyane, who led invasions into Ndau areas of central Mozambique in the convulsions of the Mfecane (Shaka Zulu's expansion north from South Africa), that caused illness and misfortune in years past. Some reported powerful spirits used for curing near the Zimbabwe border that derived from Ndebele warriors who were killed when they invaded the Shona speaking region of Manica that straddles the border. In contemporary Chimoio, as reported earlier by the author, a specific category of avenging spirit called *chikwambo* emerged repeatedly in illness narratives of women church recruits, and one pastor referred to a *chikwambo* "epidemic" in Chimoio.[33] One set of *chikwambo* spirits was repeatedly mentioned by healers, prophets, and church members: those of migrant workers who had returned to Manica from Zimbabwe or South Africa with money and goods, and had been robbed and killed upon arrival.[34] These malevolent shades are the spirits of innocent people who have been maliciously robbed and murdered and who then seek revenge on members of the killer's family, sometimes generations later, causing accidents, illness, loss of work, financial calamity, and general misfortune. In order to appease such an avenging spirit, affected families must pay the spirit back, offering young daughters to become "spirit wives," *mukadzi we mupfukwa* in Chiteve, or *mulheres de espírito* in Portuguese.[35] A spirit wife will often remain in her parents' home, although she may have children and live together with another male partner, or have many sexual partner. If the spirit wife gives birth, the children belong to the spirit as compensation and cannot be claimed by the biological father. If behavior by the wife angers the spirit, he can cause infertility, illness, and death. *Mupfukwa* spirits, including *chikwambo*, can also be harnessed by skilled curandeiros for a fee and sent to cause harm to one's enemies, a reportedly common practice among *drogados*.

The Professionalization of Healing: AMETRAMO

Many curandeiros in the city belong to the government-sponsored Mozambique Association of Traditional Healers, known by the Portuguese acronym AMETRAMO, responsible for collecting taxes and fees and setting price guidelines for services offered. An official, two-page table typed on AMETRAMO letterhead enumerates dozens of treatments and their legal prices. The table uses local spirit categories and terms in Chiteve appropriate to the city, while prices are listed for treatments that help one obtain employment, avoid accidents, contact ancestor spirits, and address a range of other common life worries and desires. Designed to control prices, the list confirms just how expensive consultations and exorcisms have become. For example, removal of a *mupfukwa* spirit costs 350,000 *meticais* (not including the initial diagnosis consultation), equivalent to nearly half a month's wages for an average worker.

A number of curandeiros, however, are distrustful of the organization and believe it exists merely to tax healers. A number of informants in the community argued that "real" (*verdadeiro*, the term used in Portuguese) curandeiros are not AMETRAMO members and can only be found in rural areas, and existence of the price list is seen by some as an indication of the organization's spuriousness. Upon leaving the home of a well-known curandeiro interviewed for this research, the local research assistant, who lives in a Chimoio *bairro*, whispered, "He's not a real curandeiro, not with a nice cement house like that, with furniture and a motorcycle." The healer's accumulation and good life were evidence that he was a fake. The 30 interviews with other residents who were not church members tended to confirm that high fees were often paid to healers and that the perception of inflated fees is widespread, and not merely an accusation made by churches.

Healing sessions for two non-church clients observed by the author provide a glimpse of the kind of problems, treatments, and fees apparently common to curandeiro practice. Not surprisingly, these sessions would not have included the dangerous practices mentioned above since the healer was being observed by an outsider. In the first case, the young male help seeker's affliction had manifested itself through a series of mishaps (especially an accident injuring his knee), misfortunes (problems at his workplace in Chimoio), and recurrent health problems (frequent trouble breathing). He had come to believe that these problems must be linked through a spiritual cause and had decided to consult the traditional healer. During the initial consultation, the curandeira contacted her personal healing spirit, who revealed himself in a deep, distinct voice and conversed directly with the young man to diagnose the problem. The healer determined that a competitor at his workplace wanted his job and had consulted another curandeiro to arrange a *mufukwa* spirit to afflict him.

To complicate matters, the help seeker's father had recently died. The curandeira indicated that this paternal spirit had withdrawn his protection for his son out of anger because the young man, the eldest son, had not conducted the annual honorific ceremony on the anniversary of the father's death. The curandeira then asked the paternal spirit for patience while she exorcized the demon sent by the man's co-worker. The process of exorcism was initiated later that day but would take several days or weeks and repeated visits to complete. The patient was advised that it might involve confronting the perpetrator at work as well. He was given a steam bath and a razor was used to make small incisions on his chest, into which *mutombo* was placed for ongoing protection. At the finish of the first day the healer asked for 350,000 *meticais* to cover the exorcism and displayed a copy of the AMETRAMO price list, which she kept in her house, to justify the high fee. In a second consultation observed by the author, another male patient complained of persistent agonizing pain in his lower leg. The curandeira quickly ascertained again, through possession by her curing spirit, that a co-worker had used sorcery powers to place several sharp pieces of wood in the man's leg to cause ongoing pain. After a lengthy period of preparation, the curandeira used her mouth to suck the items out of the patient's leg, removed the pieces from her mouth and showed them to the patient, asked for her fee, and recommended that the patient return to arrange further protection.

Given the secretive nature of the activities, it is impossible to obtain accurate information on how many people consult curandeiros and whether any change has occurred in recent years. But when interviewed for this research, the Chimoio president of AMETRAMO lamented the huge loss of business among his membership, which he attributed to the new churches. He indicated that practice of sorcery to harm others is grounds for being expelled from AMETRAMO, but he acknowledged that some curandeiros are involved.

Patterns of Resort: Money, Spirits, and Healing in the Churches

In interviews with recent church converts, prophets, and pastors, the theme of payment and legitimacy of treatment repeatedly emerged. But help-seekers also complained that curandeiros incite conflict within families and between neighbors, and then demand huge payments to take out offending spirits and provide ongoing protection from spirit threats derived from these conflicts. Most conversion stories include extended periods of help-seeking, often for both parent and child health complaints. Church membership is often the latest stop in a long sequence of seeking help for persistent afflictions such as illness, job loss, money loss, child health problems, and marital difficulties that are often perceived to be linked and caused by a single malign spirit, frequently a *chikwambo*.

Importantly, a rich and diverse range of healing repertoires, styles, ceremonies, and rituals was observed in Chimoio churches during this research. The initial healing processes conducted by many prophets, and some pastors, are similar to those of curandeiros in certain respects, suggesting the "syncretism" many observers have reported, but other aspects provide a striking and critical contrast. In some cases, prophet healers met privately at first with newcomers to divine the nature of the spiritual affliction with the help of the Holy Spirit in a manner reminiscent of curandeiro spirit possession during first consultations. The Holy Spirit acting through the prophet could identify the afflicting spirit; determine the source of the problem, often using local spirit terms; and then begin to drive the spirit out, a process that can take days to achieve. In obvious contrast to traditional healing, church pastors and prophets insist that an offending/evil spirit can only be driven out by the Holy Spirit if the help-seeker becomes a member of the church and conforms to Christian life accordingly.

While the process is sometimes initiated in private consultations to diagnose the problem, the actual exorcism of the spirit takes time and normally requires several days of fasting with others on a nearby mountain, combined with collective prayer, laying on of hands during church services, and a variety of idiosyncratic ceremonies that may include steam baths and enemas. Churches services on Sundays are normally joyous occasions with dancing, singing, and ecstatic spirituality familiar to Pentecostalism around the world. Collective baptism in nearby rivers is often included in a usually raucous, physical, and exhausting ritual process. Normally, a prophet or a pastor will eventually declare that a new member has succeeded in cleansing the spirit away. The new recruit is counseled that they must remain faithful and active in the church, however, or the Holy Spirit will withdraw its protection and the affliction will return. In important contrast with curandeiro practices, church help seekers are never advised to confront or challenge a neighbor, coworker, or family member who may have sent harm their way. Healing does not require the help seeker to engage in the often disruptive and sometimes dangerous social conflicts that may underlie afflictions. And payment is normally not requested for the prophet's services, nor is it required for the critical continuing security and protection provided by the Holy Spirit. The church healing processes center on collective action that includes continued social support and mutual aid believed to represent the generosity of the Holy Spirit.

Isabel's story of affliction, help seeking, and her decision to enter a church is typical and worth describing at some length here. She had joined a locally-founded church called *Nyasha DzaMwari* in Chiteve, or *Igreja Apostolica Graça a Deus de Moçambique* in Portuguese (The Apostolic Church Thanks to God of Mozambique) about three years before the interview. She had been raised as a Catholic in Chimoio, but a series of misfortunes and health problems provoked a sequence of help-seeking choices that ended with fasting and exorcism in the church.

> When I entered this church I had a problem with a bad spirit that was killing my daughter. I went to the hospital when my daughter got sick. My daughter didn't get better because that spirit took away the

power of the medicine [*levava aquele medicamento*] in the hospital. I had to come to this church. So, here when I arrived, he [the pastor] said this child has a bad spirit and you have to take it out. You have to go to the mountain for three days without eating anything nor drinking water to see if your daughter survives or not.

[My health problems] began a long time ago when I was a child. I always had this problem. ... I didn't marry, I got really skinny, every day I dreamt of bad things, I didn't want to go to school because of that spirit. At times I didn't even want to take a bath, I only wanted to fight with people, get insulted with people when they did nothing because that spirit gave bad luck [*azares*] in whatever way. I did manage to get married, but my husband that married me, he worked out but my spirit always abused my husband. He began to drink and he lost his job [he had been a school teacher] ... I went to the curandeiro but it wasn't possible ... The curandeiro spoke of the same things [as the church]. 'You have a bad spirit' but he didn't manage to take it out, he just took my money. The curandeiro said that this bad spirit comes from your grandparents that provoked, killed someone a long time ago ... I conceived a child who was always sick and I went many times [to the curandeiro], but now when I began to pray in these churches I saw that going to curandeiros isn't good because I always went to curandeiros and some would say pay a million *meticais* others 500,000 *meticais*. I saw that that isn't worth it. I had to come here and pray, since coming here to Nyasha DzaMwari I don't have problems and I don't go to the curandeiro anymore.

In Isabel's narrative, the curandeiro she consults provides the oft-heard description of a *chikwambo* spirit that has afflicted her for so long. She quotes the healer:

"I'm seeing this and that, I see a spirit that is chasing you but you haven't provoked anyone. Who provoked this spirit are your grandparents. A long time ago this person came from Zimbabwe and had lots of things, so your grandfather killed that person and took those blankets and things. So the spirit of that person who was killed is in your body . . . that spirit is returning to the grandchildren because the grandparents have died, so that spirit is continuing to harass you and you're suffering because of this." To end this problem you have to pay a lot of money to curandeiros. You have to bring 500,000 for him to make the spirit go away, but it never works.

Isabel's story is typical of many illness narratives as she describes seeking help at the hospital for both herself and her daughter, and continual frustration when illness returns.

> I went to the hospital, in the hospital it helped at times, they said you don't have anything what is your problem and I began to explain that I feel headaches, at times my back hurts, at times my ribs hurt, so they said let's take X-rays, they took them and said your back is okay, but they didn't know that that spirit comes at night and beats me and the next day I feel the pain. I took my child [to the hospital] I made a consultation and they said go do an analysis, I arrived there, did the analysis, then they said this child has malaria and I complied with everything there. My child, after one week or a few days, got sick again ...

She comes to see her problems with her husband as linked through spiritual affliction to these persistent health problems. The pastor's success at removing the spirit is finally manifested through her husband's new job and her own success at local petty trading.

> I had many problems, with children and with me, my husband was drinking a lot and didn't have a job, he just drank. He never contributed to expenses or anything. When he got some money he just drank in the kiosques [small neighborhood bars]. ... Because I was doing so badly I always heard and asked about a church called Nyasha dzaMwari. There they have a prophet, when you arrive there if you have a bad spirit they will take it out and you get better, so I began to ask where is this church? ... when I arrived there the pastor told me these things, he said to end all this you have to pray and this spirit will flee ... I have three years [in the church] and up to now I haven't had any problem. My husband goes to work, he brings home food, I am also working without problems.

Others who described their help-seeking and conversion experiences provided similar accounts of their involvement with curandeiros and the problem of payment. In examining the narratives of lay members, however, the meaning of monetary payment to the legitimacy of spiritual treatments emerged as a key theme in decisions, as the following selections help illustrate:

When you go to the curandeiro one pays a lot of money, but here [in the church] one doesn't pay any money. You can fast, pray to God, and your money stays with you. [Woman, Apostolic Faith Mission]

I went to the church to pray, I saw that to stay at home without praying wasn't helping and when you pray you find a lot of family, your family with the church family, you can get sick, and everyone comes to visit you, so you get a lot of family in the church. ... I can see now that the church is helping more than when I spent money going to the curandeiro to do I don't know what. I was spending a lot of money at the curandeiro. ... 1000 times I'd rather be in the church than spend money for the curandeiro. [Woman, Graça Biblica]

When you go to a curandeiro it's 600,000, 700,000 *meticais* ... just to lie, even for just 50,000 *meticais*. Because of this people are fleeing. A mother that doesn't work, doesn't do anything [for money] makes a consultation with a healer and pays 50,000, just for a fever. Because of this people are fleeing [curandeiros]. [Woman, Apostolic Faith Mission]

Curandeiros always lie that you were born sick, afterward you go there, he says I'll cure you, but you return home, you continue to be sick, a child dies, another child gets sick and dies, so you have to go to the curandeiro spending money without any result. [Man, Zion Christian Church]

Bound together with these concerns over payment is a widely shared distrust of curandeiros for the conflict they can incite with their diagnoses and recommended remedies. In interview after interview respondents commented on the dangers that curandeiros pose to social and family life. The following selections from interviews are representative.

Curandeiros are not good because they ruin the family, ruin the home, ruin everything ... They destroy, when you arrive there and they tell you that the person doing sorcery against you is so and so, if it happens to be your brother, then you believe this and you have to get your nerve up, as soon as you see that brother you get into a conflict [*fica com barulho*], because of this curandeiros are not good. [Man, Zion Christian Church]

I can go to the curandeiro and he'll say, senhor Rungo you're sick and the person doing this to you is your wife, and then love ends. I can give other examples. I arrive there, he says you're sick because your mother did this to you and I start having a conflict with my mother.

To avoid this we have to believe in Christ. With the curandeiro, you lose money, lose your family, and you lose support. [Man, Apostolic Church of Mozambique]

The curandeiro said things that aren't good, he said things that when you see your neighbor you'll fight, when in fact that's not the problem. Now in the church there isn't any of that. The church just treats you until you're cured. [Woman, Zion Apostle of Mozambique]

The problem is with curandeiros. Because we don't prohibit medicines, I go to the hospital and they have medicines there and pills and I don't know what else. If he says look you have a wound here take this medicine and you will get better. We can go to the curandeiro but he doesn't talk like that, he begins to say "come here and tell me about your life." So and so hates your family, hates you and gave you this wound. You have to separate from this family or leave that house. ... With problems with your neighbor, it comes from that house and you have to resolve the problem with your neighbor family, or whatever family, your wife's family. Your family doesn't like your wife, because of this you're sick ... [B]ecause of this our policy is we don't go to the curandeiro. [Pastor, Zion Christian Church]

Money and Healing in the Churches: "We're Poor, We Come to God Without Paying"

The circulation of money in the churches plays a crucial and complex role in the social life of the congregations, but functions very differently from payments made to curandeiros. Church contributions, in principle, are believed by lay-members to support the membership and are described as a form of redistribution; they are not linked directly to healing practices, nor are they considered payment for such help. Money in many congregations, however, also constitutes an ever-present, lurking danger that continually threatens to destabilize the collective. Many non-Pentecostals in the community are skeptical of the recent church proliferation and believe that entrepreneurial pastors recognize the potential to make money and found new churches for profit or to gain sexual access to women. A majority of the 25 pastors interviewed for this project were otherwise unemployed. Some of those interviewed believed that pastors drew in believers, especially women, through free treatment, but then extracted funds slowly over time through tithes and contributions. The international Pentecostals, such as *Reino de Deus*, or Kingdom of God, are reported to require especially high contributions from their members. All churches interviewed in this research requested financial support from their members, in some cases through regular tithing, called *dizimos* in Portuguese, to generate church funds. In Sunday service collections a hat or basket is normally passed and members are asked to donate 1,000 *meticais* if they have it, though many do not. In most cases, collections during church services are handed to a church functionary in full view of the congregation, and the total is announced. The congregation breaks into song at that moment to celebrate the generousness and solidarity of the collective as a manifestation of the Holy Spirit.

Special requests are often made in church services for contributions to members who have recently given birth or are suffering especially debilitating illnesses. In the women's groups, financial support, however modest, is often forthcoming to those in need. One woman member said, "[W]e normally help when someone is suffering, they [women in the church] come to help with whatever they can in money. The church will take out an amount from the [church] mothers, they take the money and give it to the mother, even if it's 10-20,000 *meticais*, it's a lot. We have a lot of support." One ZCC pastor explained, "a gift is a gift that you take out for your God. That money isn't to be given to somebody [*alguém*], it's only to be used in the church, the group, if it's necessary to buy a bench, or whatever the church needs." While this mutual financial assistance appears to provide a kind of safety net for church members, the defining characteristic of a false prophet or pastor, not surprisingly, is his theft of church funds or charging of fees for treatment of health problems. Most pastors handle all transactions with extreme care to avoid appearances of impropriety. In much the same way that curandeiros who may appear to be getting wealthy are distrusted, church pastors who accumulate quickly are also suspect. The fissiparous tendency of many of the churches is often blamed on disputes over these kinds of collections, as pastors often split off to form their own new churches after accusations around theft of church funds.

In spite of these concerns, successful prophets and pastors are adept at maintaining the flow of funds while dissociating offerings from treatment to avoid the appearance of sales. They then can contrast themselves with curandeiros, whose high fees and socially harmful prescriptions are confirmations of greed and malicious intent when they sell access to occult powers. Importantly, it can be appropriate for a church member to offer a prophet an item, or even money, in a spirit of thankfulness and generosity. One prophet explained the contrast between a gift and a payment:

> The curandeiro demands payment, because where he went to get his powers he had to pay, but when you go to a prophet you don't pay anything. You go to the mountain [to fast] you don't pay. Now, spiritual power is not purchased with money, you treat a person, he gets cured, later he might feel that he wants to give me something like a shirt or some corn flour that's his choice but you can't ask him to pay.

Pastors also found theological explanations for the importance of free treatment. One pastor from Nyasha dzaMwari declared,

> He [Jesus Christ] cured people, took out the bad spirits, he took them out for free, people were saved in the same way we do it here. A person comes with difficult situations and is cured and doesn't provide any reimbursement for that help he received. And because it's free we say the person is saved thanks to God and to thank him we must pray, convert and thank God, adore your God, because he has done this for you and you came to be saved, so you have to recognize God. It's because of this that many people come here, because it's done for free
> . . .

A pastor from a Zionist church provided a similar explanation:

> We allow people to go to the hospital, but not the curandeiro. Our Bible says, come to me everyone will be saved and no one is going to pay, only by your faith. Afterwards, if a brother [of the church] goes from here to a curandeiro, he's going to have his money taken in vain. We're poor, we come to God without paying . . .

There are self-declared church prophets in Chimoio who function quite like curandeiros by charging money for baptizing help-seekers in the Holy Spirit and exorcizing evil spirits outside formal congregations. Treatment has no connection to church membership. One prophet-healer had taken the name "*Mademonio*," a Chiteve-Portuguese mixed term meaning "demons." He treated people at his home using the same tools as the Zion healers (holy water, chords or *tambus*) but he had no congregation. He claimed that since he did not ask for money he was not a curandeiro, but many of his clients indicated that payment in fact was expected. Prophets who charge fees are often dismissed as curandeiros by other church leaders; payment and what it represents is a defining evaluative criterion to determine whether a prophet healer is genuine. One pastor stated,

> There exist some prophets that work for money, whatever money. This is like a curandeiro and we have a conflict with curandeiros. For example, we receive our brothers [recruits] with a health problem, an illness, we treat them but they don't pay anything. But then a nearby curandeiro will always complain. He'll see that the person is cured but didn't pay anything in the prophet's house, then he complains that "I'm paying this and I have a paper here from AMETRAMO, etc." [referring to taxes that curandeiros pay] and that's where conflict comes from. But for us, our religion doesn't allow it, cure a person and after demand payment, because we work for God.

Payment indicates that the provider is not working with God's interests in mind, and that claims to the healing power of the Holy Spirit must be false. Clients who pay have not genuinely converted, so healing cannot be successful. One ZCC pastor stated, "a person going down that road is not praying for salvation but is just doing it for their well-being of their life and nothing more." Church pastors speak of a distinction between the world, "*o mundo*," where one pays for everything, including healing, and life inside the church. But as one pastor put it, when "one goes to God it's free and you get better. I had to leave 'the world' to go in front of Jesus ... when you pay you are no longer saying that you are with Jesus but you're in the 'world.'" Transforming the healing relationship into a sale appears to undermine the legitimacy of the healer, the client's intentions, and the healing activity itself.

Discussion

Mozambicans in this region of the country have long been integrated into commoditized economies through sale of their produce and labor in wider and often international markets. The modern world had long ago intruded into local communities in the form of new products, media, land expropriation, labor extraction, and population movements. But the economic upheaval of the last ten years marks a qualitatively different, new, and deepened commodification of social and community life, inextricably bound up with growing social disparity, insecurity, mobility, and to some degree, new fortune for some. The way in which money is exchanged and circulated in this new social environment generates the kind of envy, anxieties, and suspicions around social mobility and accumulation that traditional healers have normally addressed.

The notion of "traditional" healing is itself a product of the modernist imagination and fits well with modernization theory's dualist approach to development. The recognition of traditional healers by the World Health Organization in 1975 and the 1978 Alma Ata Primary Health Care Conference elevated healers from obscurantist "witch-doctors" to "traditional health practitioners" in the modern liberal consciousness that has oriented subsequent international health practice. Modern biomedicine and public health providers, it was suggested, would do well to involve, integrate, and train local healers to help deliver modern programs and knowledge to traditional communities. The Mozambique experience described here, and the turn to Pentecostal prophet-healers, poses challenges to this simplified but persistent dualism that has informed so much public health practice in the developing world. Traditional healing had already been substantially modified by the intrusion of the modern for some time as it responded to the convulsions of colonialism and deeper integration within wider markets over at least the last 100 years. This is evidenced by the primacy of certain spirit groups, such as *chikwambo*, that appear to emanate from the social ruptures created by labor migration to Rhodesia and South Africa and the new material inequalities they generated. In other words, "traditional" healing practices in some sense had already "modernized" and provided help-seekers with tools to navigate modern social dilemmas. The rejection of curandeiros and the turn to the Holy Spirit is most likely part of a long history of continual change and adaptation in healing practices, philosophies, and ideas in the region. Therapeutic processes, ritual forms, and types of payment for healing have likely undergone constant revision in Mozambique's complex political economic and cultural history. The current moment is an especially important one in central Mozambique, not because modernity has just arrived, but because new forms of power relations, class struggles, and market forces have jarred these communities in different ways once again. The rapid withdrawal of safety nets, growing inequality, and new pathways to accumulation that characterize this particular phase of peripheral capitalism in this specific post-colonial moment have confounded and distorted previous healing approaches and provided an opening for alternatives.

Processes of globalization and migration have made Pentecostal ideas more easily available to these communities, but that is not to say that the popularity of Pentecostals and AICs represents a new plunge into modernity or an immersion in new globalized identities. Curandeiros remain an important source of support for many Mozambicans, especially for men seeking fortune and protection. In this way, "traditional" healers remain, for some, as relevant and necessary to surviving and prospering in "modern" Chimoio as church prophets. For others, especially women, curandeiros alienate more than they heal in the new context, and the Pentecostal message brings a different and dynamic healing experience well-suited to this new marginalization. The new, local, and all-too-real micropolitics[36] of startling inequities remain the focus of help-seeking processes that are filling the churches.

Rather than situating Pentecostal success within the generalized and supposedly inevitable processes of transition from "invented" tradition to global modernity, it is argued here that the recent turn to the Holy Spirit in Mozambique underscores the social tragedy of the current free-fall free-market experiment: an experiment that was neither inevitable nor synonymous with modernity. The ongoing recalibration of traditional healing to new social environments, and the arrival of new competing healing discourses in Mozambique, provides additional evidence to support Terence Ranger's warning that "the history of modern tradition has been much more complex than we have supposed."[37]

Acknowledgements

This research has been made possible by individual research grants from the National Science Foundation (BCS-0135860) and the Wenner-Gren Foundation for Anthropological Research (Grant 6784). Additional logistic support was provided by Health Alliance International in Mozambique and the Manica Province Health Directorate.

Notes

[1]Reprinted, with permission, from *Culture, Medicine and Psychiatry* 29 (2005): 255-83.

[2]Because of overlap in central tenets and practices, and in spite of some very important differences, this paper treats AICs and Pentecostal Churches as constitutive of a general

Pentecostal movement. They are similar in their incorporation of key tenets of Pentecostalism, including belief in the healing power of the "Holy Spirit," the authority of New Testament scripture, ritualized speaking in tongues, ceremonies of baptism, and spiritual explanations for misfortune and illness (Harvey Cox, *Fire From Heaven: The Rise of Pentecostal Spirituality and the Reshaping of Religion in the Twenty First Century* (Reading, Mass.: Addison-Wesley Publishing, 1995). Both groupings of churches trace their histories to the same early Pentecostals. However, there are important differences as well. Some of the Pentecostals in Chimoio have international links to global networks, while AICs by definition are linked only to regional groups and are often founded locally. The major perceived distinction between the AICs and more mainstream Pentecostals in Chimoio is the use of prophet-healers (*profecia* in Portuguese) by AICs to communicate with the spirit world during the healing process in ways that are often called "syncretistic." For mainstream Pentecostals, such as the African Assembly of God, this prophet-healing recalls African traditional healing and is frowned upon. Instead, prayer (summoning the Holy Spirit) and laying-on of hands is used by pastors to heal. There are, however, some well-known international Pentecostals in Chimoio, such as the Apostolic Faith Mission, that have recently begun prophet-healing, perhaps as a strategy to gain more members. Two sets of AICs, the Zionists and the Apostolics, use prophetic healing. See extended discussion in James Pfeiffer, "African Independent Churches in Mozambique: Healing the Afflictions of Inequality," *Medical Anthropology Quarterly* 16 (2002): 176-199. The influence of Pentecostalist ideas among AICs can be traced historically to the arrival of Pentecostals from the U.S.-based Apostolic Faith Mission and "Zionist" evangelists from Alexander Dowie's Zion City, Illinois (who increasingly adopted Pentecostal principles) to South Africa in the early 20th century. See Cox, *Fire From Heaven*; Jean Comaroff, *Body of Power, Spirit of Resistance* (Chicago: University of Chicago Press, 1985); Bengt G. M. Sundkler, *Bantu Prophets in South Africa*, 2nd edition (London: Oxford University Press, 1961). The terms "Apostolic" and "Zion" appear in the names of many AICs, but it is often difficult to determine historical linkages because of the tendencies toward splits and local founding of new independent congregations.

[3] Pfeiffer, "African Independent Churches in Mozambique."

[4] Sundkler, *Bantu Prophets in South Africa*; Marthinus Daneel, *Zionism and Faith-Healing in Rhodesia* (The Hague: Mouton and Co., 1970); Marthinus Daneel, *Old and New in Southern Shona Independent Churches: Leadership and Fission Dynamics*, vol. 3 (Gweru, Zimbabwe: Mambo Press, 1988); Gerhardus C. Oosthuizen, *The Healer-Prophet in Afro-Christian Churches* (Leiden: E. J. Brill, 1992); Michael Bourdillon, *The Shona Peoples*, 3rd edition (Gweru, Zimbabwe: Mambo Press, 1991).

[5] See for example, James Kiernan, "Poor and Puritan: An Attempt to View Zionism as a Collective Response to Urban Poverty," *African Studies* 36 (1977): 31-41; James Kiernan, "Images of Rejection in the Construction of Morality: Satan and the Sorcerer as Moral Signposts in the Social Landscape of Urban Zionists," *Social Anthropology* 5 (1997): 243-252; Marthinus Daneel, "Exorcism as a Means of Combating Wizardry: Liberation or Enslavement", in *Empirical Studies of African Independent/Indigenous Churches*, edited by Gerhardus C. Oosthuizen and Irving Hexham, (Lewiston, New York: The EdwinMellenPress, 1992), 195-238; D. Dube, "A Search for Abundant Life: Health, Healing and Wholeness in the Zionist Churches," in *Afro-Christian Religion and Healing in Southern Africa*, ed. Gerhardus C. Oosthuizen, S.D. Edwards, W.H. Wessels and Irv-

ing Hexham (Lewiston, New York: The Edwin Mellen Press, 1989), 111-136; Gerhardus
C. Oosthuizen, "Indigenous Healing Within the Context of the African Independent
Churches," in *Afro-Christian Religion and Healing in Southern Africa*, 73-90; Sundkler,
Bantu Prophets in South Africa.
   [6]Terence Ranger, "Religious Movements and Politics in Sub-Saharan Africa," *African
Studies Review* 29 (1986): 1-69; Linda E. Thomas, "African Indigenous Churches as a
Source of Socio-Political Transformation in South Africa," *Africa Today* (1994): 39-56;
Peter Walshe, "South Africa: Prophetic Christianity and the Liberation Movement," *The
Journal of Modern South Africa* 29 (1991): 27-60; Matthew Schoffeleers, "Ritual Healing
and Political Acquiescence: The Case of the Zionist Churches in Southern Africa," *Africa*
60 (1991): 1-25; Comaroff, *Body of Power, Spirit of Resistance*.
   [7]Cf. Andre Corten, and Ruth Marshall-Fratani, eds., *Between Babel and Pentecost:
Transnational Pentecostalism in Africa and Latin America* (Bloomington, IN: Indiana
University Press, 2001); Karla Poewe, ed., *Charismatic Christianity as a Global Culture*
(Columbia, SC: University of South Carolina, 1994); Peter Van Der Veer, ed., *Conversion to Modernities: The Globalization of Christianity* (New York: Routledge, 1995);
Simon Coleman, *The Globalization of Charismatic Christianity: Spreading the Gospel
of Prosperity* (Cambridge: Cambridge University Press, 2000); Birgit Meyer, "'Make a
Complete Break with the Past:' Memory and Postcolonial Modernity in Ghanaian Pentecostal Discourse," in *Memory and the Postcolony: African Anthropology and the Critique
of Power*, ed. Richard Werbner (London: Zed Books, 1998), 182-208; Rijk Van Dijk,
"Pentecostalism, Cultural Memory and the State: Contested Representations of Time in
Postcolonial Malawi," in *Memory and the Postcolony*, 182-208.
   [8]Meyer, "Make a Complete Break with the Past."
   [9]Birgit Meyer, "'If You Are a Devil, You Are a Witch and if You Are a Witch, You
Are a Devil': The Integration of 'Pagan' Ideas into the Conceptual Universe of Ewe
Christians in Southeastern Ghana," in *Power and Prayer*, ed. Mart Bax and Adrianus
Koster (Amsterdam: V.U. University Press, 1993), 159-182.; Meyer, "Make a Complete
Break with the Past."
   [10]Max Gluckman, *Custom and Conflict in Africa* (Oxford: Basil Blackwell, 1955);
Maxwell G. Marwick, *Sorcery in its Social Setting: A Study of the Northern Rhode-
sia Cewa* (Manchester: Manchester University Press, 1965); Edward Evans-Pritchard,
Witchcraft, Oracles, and Magic among the Azande (Oxford: Clarendon Press, 1937);
John Middleton, and E.H. Winter, eds., *Witchcraft and Sorcery in East Africa* (London:
Routledge and Kegan Paul, 1963); Jean Comaroff and John Comaroff, Introduction to
Modernity and Its Malcontents: Ritual and Power in Postcolonial Africa, ed. Jean Co-
maroff and John Comaroff (Chicago: University of Chicago Press, 1993), xi-xxxvii; Peter
Geschiere, *The Modernity of Witchcraft* (Charlottesville: University Press of Virginia,
1997); Henrietta Moore and Todd Sanders, *Magical Interpretations, Material Realities:
Modernity, Witchcraft and the Occult in Postcolonial Africa* (London: Routledge, 2001).
As Moore and Sanders remind us, Evans-Pritchard's view differed from the structural-
functionalist Manchester School (Gluckman, Marwick, Turner and others) that reduced
witchcraft to a 'social strain-gauge' and pressure valve that helped maintain social home-
ostasis. See further discussion in Moore and Sanders, *Magical Interpretations, Material
Realities*, 6-13.
   [11]Peter Geschiere, "Globalization and the Power of Indeterminate Meaning: Witchcraft

and Spirit Cults in Africa and East Asia," in *Globalization and Identity: Dialectics of Flow and Closure*, ed. Birgit Meyer and Peter Geschiere (Oxford: Blackwell Publishers, 1999), 211-237.

[12]Dirk Kohnert, "Magic and Witchcraft: Implications for Democratization and Poverty-Alleviating Aid in Africa," *World Development* 24 (1996): 1347-1355; David Maxwell, "Witches, Prophets and Avenging Spirits: The Second Christian Movement in North-East Zimbabwe," *Journal of Religion in Africa* 25 (1995): 309-339; David Maxwell, "Historicizing Christian Independency: The Southern African Pentecostal Movement c. 1908-60," *Journal of African History* 40 (1999): 243-264; Geschiere, *The Modernity of Witchcraft*; Geschiere, "Globalization and the Power of Indeterminate Meaning"; Meyer, "If You Are a Devil, You Are a Witch"; Comaroff and Comaroff, Introduction to *Modernity and Its Malcontents*; Jean Comaroff and John Comaroff, "Occult Economies and the Violence of Abstraction: Notes from the South African Postcolony," *American Ethnologist* 26(1999): 279-303; Mark Auslander, "'Open the Wombs!': The Symbolic Politics of Modern Ngoni Witchfinding", in *Modernity and Its Malcontents*, ed. Jean and John Comaroff, 167-192; C. Bawa Yamba, "Cosmologies in Turmoil: Witchfinding and AIDS in Chiawa, Zambia," *Africa* 67 (1997): 200-223; Harri Englund, "Witchcraft, Modernity and the Person," *Critique of Anthropology* 16 (1996): 257-279; Moore and Sanders, *Magical Interpretations, Material Realities*; Todd Sanders, "Reconsidering Witchcraft: Postcolonial Africa and Analytic (Un)certainties," *American Anthropologist* 105 (2003): 338-352.

[13]Geschiere, "Globalization and the Power of Indeterminate Meaning," 213.

[14]See discussions in Gluckman, *Custom and Conflict in Africa*; Marwick, *Sorcery in its Social Setting*; Evans-Pritchard, *Witchcraft, Oracles, and Magic among the Azande*; and Middleton and Winter, *Witchcraft and Sorcery in East Africa*. Maxwell mentions *chikwambo* spirits in Zimbabwe, and some ethnography on Shona healing in Zimbabwe refers to *chikwambo nyangas* who are consulted by clients seeking retribution from someone who has harmed them, or failed to pay back debt. See Maxwell, "Witches, Prophets and Avenging Spirits," and Michael Gelfand, S. Mavi, R. B. Drummond, and B. Ndemera, *The Traditional Medical Practitioner in Zimbabwe* (Gweru: Mambo Press, 1985).

[15]Comaroff, and Comaroff, Introduction to *Modernity and Its Malcontents*, xxvii.

[16]Moore and Sanders, *Magical Interpretations, Material Realities*, 12, emphasis added.

[17]Sanders, "Reconsidering Witchcraft," 168.

[18]See also Rachel Chapman, "Endangering Safe Motherhood in Mozambique: Prenatal Care as Reproductive Risk," *Social Science and Medicine* 57 (2003): 355-374, for discussion on the vulnerability of pregnant women to sorcery in central Mozambique.

[19]INE (Instituto Nacional de Estatística), *Inquérito Nacional aos Agregados Familiares Sobre Condições de Vida – 1996-1997 (National Family Survey on Living Conditions)*, (Maputo: Government of Mozambique, 1998).

[20]INE (Instituto Nacional de Estatística), *II Recenseamento Geral da População e Habitação, 1997: Província de Manica (Second General Census: Manica Province)* (Maputo: Government of Mozambique, 1999).

[21]UNDP (United Nations Development Programme), *National Human Development Report on Mozambique* (Oxford: Oxford University Press, 1998).

[22]Julie Cliff, "The War on Women in Mozambique: Health Consequences of South African Destabilization, Economic Crisis, and Structural Adjustment," in *Women and*

Health in Africa, ed. Meredeth Turshen, (Trenton, N.J.: Africa World Press, 1991), 15-33.

[23]INE (Instituto Nacional de Estatística), *II Recenseamento Geral da População e Habitação*, 1997.

[24]Alex Vines and Ken Wilson, "Churches and the Peace Process in Mozambique," in *The Christian Churches and the Democratization of Africa*, ed. Paul Gifford, (Leiden: E. J. Brill., 1995), 130-147.

[25]Judith Marshall, "Structural Adjustment and Social Policy in Mozambique," *Review of African Political Economy* 17 (1990): 28-43; Cliff, "The War on Women in Mozambique"; Joseph Hanlon, *Peace Without Profit: How the IMF Blocks Rebuilding in Mozambique* (Oxford: James Currey, 1996).

[26]Paul Fauvet, "Mozambique: Growth with Poverty, A Difficult Transition from Prolonged War to Peace and Development" *Africa Recovery* 14 (2000): 1; Hanlon, *Peace Without Profit.*

[27]Ministry of Planning and Finance, Mozambique, *Understanding Poverty and Well-Being in Mozambique: The First National Assessment (1996-97)* (Maputo: Government of Mozambique, 1998); Hanlon, *Peace Without Profit*; INE (Instituto Nacional de Estatística), *Inquérito Nacional aos Agregados Familiares Sobre Condições de Vida – 1996-1997.*

[28]See similar findings in Ministry of Planning and Finance, *Understanding Poverty and Well-Being in Mozambique*, 312.

[29]James Pfeiffer, Stephen Gloyd, and Lucy Ramierez Li, "Intrahousehold Resource Allocation and Child Growth in Central Mozambique: An Ethnographic Case-Control Study," *Social Science & Medicine* 53 (2001): 83-97.

[30]G. L. Chavunduka, *Traditional Healers and the Shona Patient* (Gwelo: Mambo Press, 1978); Michael Gelfand, *Shona Religion (With Special Reference to the Korekore)* (Cape Town: Juta, 1962); Gelfand, Mavi, Drummond, and Ndemera, *The Traditional Medical Practitioner in Zimbabwe*; and Bourdillon, *The Shona Peoples.*

[31]Pfeiffer, "African Independent Churches in Mozambique"; Chavunduka, *Traditional Healers and the Shona Patient*; David Lan, *Guns and Rain: Guerillas and Spirit Mediums in Zimbabwe* (London: James Currey, 1985); Gelfand, *Shona Religion*; and Bourdillon, *The Shona Peoples.*

[32]Cf. Bourdillon, *The Shona Peoples*, and Lan, *Guns and Rain*, for descriptions of similar spirits called *ngozi* in Zimbabwe.

[33]Pfeiffer, "African Independent Churches in Mozambique."

[34]In "Witches, Prophets and Avenging Spirits," Maxwell mentions *chikwambo* spirits in Zimbabwe, and some ethnography on Shona healing in Zimbabwe refers to *chikwambo nyangas* who are consulted by clients seeking retribution for someone who has harmed them, or failed to pay back debt. See Gelfand, Mavi, Drummond, and Ndemera, *The Traditional Medical Practitioner in Zimbabwe.*

[35]See also discussion in Chapman, "Endangering Safe Motherhood in Mozambique."

[36]Comaroff and Comaroff, Introduction to *Modernity and Its Malcontents.*

[37]Terence Ranger, "The Invention of Tradition Revisited: The Case of Colonial Africa," in *Legitimacy and the State in Twentieth-Century Africa*, ed. Terence Ranger and Olufeni Vaughan (London: Macmillan, 1993), 62-111.

CHAPTER 12

The Long Shadow of Colonialism: Why We Study Medicine in Africa

JONATHAN SADOWSKY

Shortly before the Bryn Mawr Workshop on Health and Medicine in Africa, I attended a public lecture at my own university, where I met an undergraduate student sitting near me. She was bright and argumentative, so I tried to encourage her to take an African history class with me. She declined, noting that she had already taken an African history course at another school. When I asked her how she liked the course, she said that while she found it illuminating to learn of the horrors of colonialism, she believed that much went unsaid because of "political correctness." When I asked for an example, she replied that it was, after all, better to have penicillin than not. This comment struck me as at once true in a sense, but also revealing about a historical memory of colonialism still powerful in the West: the image of colonialism as a Schweitzer-like figure dispensing medicines to people who lacked medical care.

As the study of medicine in Africa has grown over the last 25 years, a lot of scholarship has helped to complicate this image. Even leaving aside the efficacy of traditional African medicines, we now know that during the colonial period discrimination against African doctors (even those with biomedical training) grew,[1] that colonial medical services were often designed to serve the health of the colonial state and economic projects as much, if not more than, the bodies of African subjects,[2] that social changes wrought by colonialism could be a major contributor to ill-health,[3] and that colonial medical science could be fruitfully read as an ideological artifact of colonial domination.[4] Schweitzer himself was, in deep and significant ways, an expression of colonial values and assumptions.[5] Yet, this student's enduring image came after taking an African history course, and was based on presumptions on what must have been suppressed in her instructors account. This suggests we have a lot more work to do – not just research work, but work towards thinking through our messages and how to communicate them, an agenda that was carried forward in the Bryn Mawr conference in productive ways. This essay builds on an oral commentary I gave at that conference. Since my panel was one of the first, I commented not only on the papers presented, but also ventured an overview of the conference's claims to significance, and concluded with a suggestion on what social studies of medicine in Africa might communicate to scholars in related areas.

The conference's significance, I thought, could be based on at least four observations.[6] The first is evident in the exchange with the student mentioned above: the role of medicine in Western memory of colonialism. The second one is the reverse: the role of Western medicine in African historical memory. African distrust of biomedical institutions is rooted not simply in cultural difference, but in concrete historical experience.[7] Thirdly, medicine has an unusual ability to cast light simultaneously on the social structural and the intimate, to allow us to see the social forces that produce suffering, and the personal bodily experiences of the suffering. While true of medicine everywhere, this takes on special significance in Africa, because of the severity of the contemporary medical crises there, and the ways they both reflect and aggravate the political crises. And finally, there is medicine's often-noted role as justification for imperialism.

The panel in which I served as discussant featured the papers by Webb, Pfeiffer and Ngalamulume, included in this collection. On one level, the topics were enormously diverse: one on the very early history of human encounter with infectious disease in Africa, one on a colonial institution intended to manage mental illness in the early colonial period, and one on contemporary transformations in the social organization of healing. Yet despite their topical and temporal breadth, there is a common thread running through them. All the papers (and indeed, all the papers in the conference) are shadowed by the violence – physical, social-structural, and epistemological – of colonialism. Since the end of the colonial period, African studies scholars have debated the merits of using colonialism as a central organizing principle for periodizing the African past. There is, for example, a danger of over-stating Western influence on Africa, or in other words, under-stating African agency.[8] As Margaret Field noted in her study of mental illness in late colonial Ghana, this approach also risks over-stressing the significance of the state.[9] While recognizing the power of these arguments, Africa's continuing economic and political challenges encourage an emphasis on colonialism, because it is hard to make sense of those challenges without this emphasis.[10] Colonialism had deep and lasting effects on the structures of knowledge, and its policies continue to influence the course of contemporary Africa. Seeing the shadow colonialism casts over the very different research agendas discussed here strengthens this argument.

In the case of James Webb's enormously ambitious research, that shadow is seen in the form of what I am calling epistemological violence. In trying to reconstruct critical aspects of the early African, and human past, Webb needs to look not directly at it, but through the colonial period, and the assumptions about Africa and Africans generated by racism. While dealing with many other important themes, Webb's contribution illustrates the significance of this colonial prism in at least two ways. The first is his replacement of a Eurocentric model of the rise of "modern" human behavior with one that locates critical changes in social and economic organization in African history. The second is his dislodging of the assumption that the migrations of Bantu-speaking peoples took place through processes of violent invasion and conquest. According to this assumption, the spread of African peoples through the continent was assumed, despite slender evidence, to have followed the very pattern of the arrival of Europeans during the modern colonial era.

In my oral commentary at the workshop, I went further than this, challenging Webb to find traces of epistemological violence in the contemporary science that he treated as superseding the science compromised by colonial assumptions. In what I took to be a response to this challenge (as well, perhaps, to other aspects of my commentary) Helen Tilley raised the concern that too expansive a use of the term "violence" risks debasing the word altogether, rendering it meaningless. Her well-taken point relates to a larger and important reminder that science in colonial (and post-colonial) contexts needs to be seen not only as a reflection or tool of empire, but as a source of useful knowledge that could be used in progressive and even anti-colonial ways. The phrase "epistemological violence" may be an accurate enough description of scientific racism, but if we are automatically suspicious of any and all science, or question any claims to scientific advance by debunking them as "progress narratives" in a knee-jerk fashion, why do any research at all? Why, for example, engage in social studies of science, if we had no hope it could yield better science? These questions in turn suggest another way of looking at the conversation with a student with which I began. Perhaps one way of improving the ways we tell the history of medicine in Africa is to do so with these ambiguities firmly in mind. The student, in other words, may not have been calling simply for a more benevolent story of colonialism, but for a more complicated one.

Kalala Ngalamulume's paper adds to our knowledge of colonial psychiatric institutions, and contributes to our ability to make systematic comparisons. It is striking, for example, that in much of colonial Africa, urban "madness" emerged as a policy problem in the 1890s. As Ngalamulume shows, this is likely less a symptom of any increase in psychopathology, than a symptom of a particular stage in the development of the colonial state, a stage where questions of state responsibility were beginning to be asked, assuming new significance as colonialism began an uneven transition from a mode of conquest to a mode of administration. Ngalamulume's paper also reinforces our awareness that the medical records of colonial psychiatric institutions often provided very scant evidence of illness. We therefore have a warrant to read them critically, to wonder what role cultural incomprehension or political difference had in the confinement and diagnosis of the individual. We should not, however, be too quick to assume that the person was not ill in some meaningful sense. But even if we take the person to be ill, we can be alert to what specific symptom or trait was noted in these cursory records, as a possible clue to what was disturbing or striking to the people responsible for the confinement. In Ngalamulume's work, this is most clearly seen in the extended discussion of the patient Jules and the apparent gulf between his perceptions and those of the people who confined him.

In James Pfeiffer's paper, we see the medical and health effects for a society emerging from a brutal series of late colonial and post-colonial conflicts, compounded by contemporary neo-liberalism and structural adjustment. I first read Pfeiffer's paper at the same time as I was reading Eli Zaretsky's remarkable history of psychoanalysis, and was struck by similarities between the decline in popularity of psychoanalysis and that of the *curandeiros*.[11] Zaretsky argues that psychoanalysis flourished when it was the appropriate modality for a given social and economic context (the second or Fordist, industrial revolution in the West) and declined when that context passed.[12] Like the psychoanalysts, the *curandeiros* increasingly priced themselves out of the market during a period when large numbers of people were struggling to pay for health care, and so like the psychoanalysts have lost customers to new providers (in the case of the analysts, mainly psychopharmaceutical providers).

This comparison runs the risk of being stretched too far. I make it, though, for two reasons. For one, while reading Pfeiffer, I wondered whether the decline of the *curandeiros* might entail a loss of valuable knowledge (if you believe, as I do, that psychoanalysis has something to offer, its social decline is cause for at least some concern along these lines). We do know that, apart from any tendencies to romanticize traditional healers in Africa, there have been robust healing traditions that were not just culturally and symbolically powerful, but efficacious in ways closer to what is explicitly valued by cosmopolitan biomedicine.[13] Secondly, I wonder if the comparison may help lead to broader comparisons of medical (and social) changes between North America and Africa. Barbara Ehrenreich has, for example, argued that Evangelical churches increasingly derive much of their power from a growing role as social service providers – a role that both profits from a dwindling welfare state, and contributes to it.[14] In the United States, as well, the state's ability to provide social welfare is declining in a context of growing economic inequality. There are, of course, enormous differences between the African and North American contexts, but perhaps the commonalities can help illuminate patterned relationships between religious institutions and neo-liberalism, reflecting global trends with effects that are in some ways parallel, though significantly different.

My conclusion begins with another anecdote. I once attended a panel on "Colonies" at the annual meeting of the American Association for the History of Medicine. The room was packed for a paper on colonial New England but became gradually emptier as the papers grew less relevant to the study of the United States. The final paper was about South Africa and was poorly attended. This was at once understandable (most members of the AAHM are Americanists), and frankly annoying. But while it is appropriate to criticize any ethnocentrism and parochialism that may have been present, I also wonder what we, as students of health and medicine in Africa, could do to communicate better with our colleagues, to persuade them of our significance, to highlight the general relevance of our work.

One possibility would be to use our knowledge of colonial medicine to complicate the "colonial" metaphor that historians of medicine have sometimes used to describe medicine in modernity. We frequently see descriptions of modern medicine as "colonizing" ever more spheres of life, where colonization is used as a metaphorical synonym for medicalization. As I have argued elsewhere,[15] there is some irony in this, since what is distinctive about colonial medicine (and by extension, colonial policies) in many contexts is its neglect, its irresponsible distance from even the sick. Perhaps this is the main point: what was colonial about colonial medicine was that it was as invasive and coercive as modern medicine could be, but insufficiently therapeutic and supportive to warrant the invasion.

As Julie Livingston argued eloquently at the Bryn Mawr conference, historians of medicine might profit from the study of African epistemologies and ethos. Livingston made this point by drawing attention to the emphasis, in many African conceptions, on medicine's knife-edge ability to both heal and harm. Harm done by medicine may be recognized as a possibility in Western cultures, but is usually thought to be anomalous, leaving Western societies with few culturally palatable means of managing it and understanding it. In making this point, Livingston argued that the growing interest in the study of patients, as a corrective to previous over-emphasis on clinicians, carries its own dangers of over-emphasis. For those historians of medicine, though, who are interested in "the patient's perspective," there may also be much to be learned from the ways Africa scholars have complicated the notion of "African voices," and the increasing awareness in recent scholarship that there is not one single African perspective.[16] In a classic article about patient-centered history of medicine, Roy Porter seemed to assume that the voice of the patient would be a unified voice of resistance to the dominance of the physician, a corrective to medicine's most idealized self-image.[17] This assumption evokes, for an Africa scholar, the representation of African perspectives as unified voices of resistance to colonialism, a common trope in African studies from the 1960s and 1970s. This was itself a colonial assumption, in at least two ways: it reified the African subject, and made colonialism the center of that subject's preoccupations – perhaps even reifying colonialism itself. More recent scholarship, such as the work presented at the Bryn Mawr conference, has shown emphatically that there is not one Africa, not a single "African subject." Nor was there one colonialism; the shadow of colonialism may be long, but it is uneven. The idea of a monolithic "African voice" therefore also reflected a simplistic view of colonialism, and of power itself.

Notes

[1]See, for example, Adell Patton, Jr., *Physicians, Colonial Racism, and Diaspora in West Africa* (Gainesville: University of Florida, 1996).

[2]See, for example, Megan Vaughan, *Curing Their Ills: Colonial Power and African Illness* (Stanford: Stanford University, 1991); George O. Ndege, *Health, State, and Society in Kenya* (Rochester, NY: University of Rochester Press, 2001).

[3]See, for example, Maryinez Lyons, *A Colonial Disease: A Social History of Sleeping Sickness in Northern Zaire, 1900-1940* (Cambridge: Cambridge University Press, 1992).

[4]See, for example, Vaughan, *Curing Their Ills*; Randall Packard, "The 'Healthy Reserve' and the 'Dressed Native': Discourses on Black Health and the Language of Legitimation in South Africa," *American Ethnologist* 16 (1989): 686-703; Jock McCulloch, *Colonial Psychiatry and the African Mind* (Cambridge: Cambridge University, 1995).

[5]See my review of new editions of Schweitzer's writings in *Bulletin of the History of Medicine* 74, 2 (2000): 394-396.

[6]These could, of course, be added to at length.

[7]Jonathan Sadowsky, *Imperial Bedlam: Institutions of Madness and Colonialism in Southwest Nigeria* (Berkeley: University of California Press, 1999), 116.

[8]This seems, for example, to be one implication of J. F. A. Ajayi, "The Continuity of African Institutions under Colonialism," in *Emerging Themes of African History*, ed. Terence Ranger (Nairobi: East African Publishing House, 1968).

[9]Margaret Field, *Search for Security: An Ethnopsychiatric Study of Rural Ghana* (London: Faber & Faber, 1960).

[10]One of the best statements of this view is Crawford Young, *The African Colonial State in Comparative Perspective* (New Haven: Yale University, 1994). As Young shows in exhaustive detail, the specific features of the colonial state in Africa – the ways it differed from other modern colonial states – continue to vex Africa's prospects.

[11]Eli Zaretsky, *Secrets of the Soul: A Social and Cultural History of Psychoanalysis* (New York: Alfred A. Knopf, 2004).

[12]For Zaretsky, psychoanalysis provided the cultural organization for an emerging concept of personal life specific to Fordism, just as in Max Weber's famous formulation, Calvinism was an apt cultural expression of an earlier form of capitalism.

[13]I make this argument in relation to Yoruba mental healing: Jonathan Sadowsky, "Confinement and Colonialism in Nigeria," in *The Confinement of the Insane, 1800-1965: International Perspectives*, ed. Roy Porter and David Wright (Cambridge, Cambridge University Press, 2003), 300.

[14]Barbara Ehrenreich, "The Faith Factor," *The Nation*, November 29, 2004, also available at http://www.thenation.com/doc/20041129/ehrenreich. Ehrenreich writes, "What these churches have to offer, in addition to intangibles like eternal salvation, is concrete, material assistance. They have become an alternative welfare state, whose support rests not only on 'faith' but also on the loyalty of the grateful recipients."

[15]Sadowsky, "Confinement and Colonialism," 313-314.

[16]See, for example, Luise White, *Speaking with Vampires: Rumor and History in Colo-*

nial Africa. Berkeley (University of California Press, 2000), and David William Cohen and E. S. Atieno Odhiambo, *The Risks of Knowledge: Investigations into the Death of the Ho. Minister John Robert Ouko in Kenya, 1990* (Athens: Ohio University Press, 2004).

[17] Roy Porter, "The Patient's View: Doing Medical History from Below," *Theory and Society* 14 (1985): 175-198. This is an old article, however great and influential its author was, and cannot be used to stand in for an entire field – but I do believe that thinking about the meaning of the patient's perspective in medical history would profit from more of the kind of explicit discussion that the meaning of African voices has received.